QUALITY O

Concern about the quality of life and its measurement is probably greater now than ever before. Economists investigating health care have recognised the need to develop outcome measures. Social scientists have tried to address whether or not government intervention has improved the welfare of the relevant client group. The government itself in emphasising the need for programmes to be cost-effective has provoked researchers to attempt to find acceptable definitions and empirical measures of quality of life that can be used in policy debates.

The issues addressed in this volume range from the philosophical question of what the good life is to detailed studies of what constitutes a good quality of life for particular client groups; from technical discussion of the features of a quality of life measure to scrutiny of the difficult, and possibly controversial, implications of using such a measure as part of the resource allocation process.

Researchers from traditionally separate disciplines are being forced to confront similar issues and this collection highlights the benefits of linking the experiences of applied researchers, those engaged in theoretical debate, and those engaged in policy analysis. *Quality of Life* will be valuable reading for researchers and practitioners in social policy, social work and economics.

The editors
Sally Baldwin is the Director of the Social Policy Research Unit at the University of York; Christine Godfrey is a Senior Research Fellow in the Centre for Health Economics, also at the University of York: Carol Propper is a lecturer in the School of Advanced Urban Studies and the Department of Economics at Bristol University.

QUALITY OF LIFE

Perspectives and Policies

EDITED BY SALLY BALDWIN,
CHRISTINE GODFREY AND
CAROL PROPPER

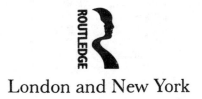

London and New York

First published 1990
Reprinted 1991, 1992 by Routledge
11 New Fetter Lane, London EC4P 4EE

Simultaneously published in the USA and Canada
by Routledge
a division of Routledge, Chapman and Hall, Inc.
29 West 35th Street, New York, NY 10001

First published in paperback by
Routledge in 1994

Printed and bound in Great Britain by
Biddles Ltd, Guildford and King's Lynn

British Library Cataloguing in Publication Data

Quality of life: perspectives and policies.
1. Quality of life
I. Baldwin, Sally   II. Godfrey, Christine
III. Propper, Carol, *1956*–
303

Library of Congress Cataloging in Publication Data

Quality of Life: perspectives and policies / edited by Sally Baldwin,
Christine Godfrey, and Carol Propper.
p.   cm.
Includes bibliographical references and indexes.
1. Quality of life–Congresses.   I. Baldwin, Sally.   II. Godfrey,
Christine, 1950–.   III. Propper, Carol, 1956–
HN25.Q345 1994

0–415–09581–6

306–dc20

93-25921
CIP

CONTENTS

PART FOUR POLICY ISSUES

CONTRIBUTORS

Sally Baldwin   Professor, Director of Social Policy Research Unit, University of York.

Christine Godfrey   Senior Research Fellow, Centre for Health Economics, University of York.

Anthony J. Culyer   Professor, Pro Vice Chancellor, Head of Department of Economics and Related Studies, University of York.

Paul Kind   Senior Research Fellow, Centre for Health Economics, University of York.

Claire Gudex   Research Fellow, Centre for Health Economics, University of York.

Graham Loomes   Professor, Department of Economics and Related Studies, University of York.

Lynda McKenzie   18 St Ronan's Circle, Peterculter, Aberdeen.

Alan Shiell   Centre for Health Economics Research and Evaluation, Westmead and Parramatta Hospitals and Community Health Services, Westmead Hospital, NSW, Australia.

Catherine Pettipher   Department of Social Policy, University of Manchester.

Norma Raynes   Trafford Metropolitan Borough Council Social Services Department, Manchester.

Ken Wright   Deputy Director, Centre for Health Economics, University of York.

Gillian Parker   Social Policy Research Unit, University of York.

Celia Downes   Social Policy and Social Work, University of York.

Anne Corden   Research Fellow, Social Policy Research Unit, University of York.

Sandra Hutton   Research Fellow, Social Policy Research Unit, University of York.

Melanie Powell   Lecturer, Department of Economics, University of Leeds.

Alan Maynard   Professor, Director, Centre for Health Economics, University of York.

Alison Eastwood   Division of Health Policy, Research and Education, Harvard University, Boston, Massachusetts.

Carol Propper   Lecturer, Department of Economics, University of Bristol.

Chris Megone   Department of Philosophy, University of Leeds.

Joanna Hodge   Faculty of Humanities, Law and Social Science, Department of Inter-Disciplinary Studies, Manchester Polytechnic.

Karen Gerard   Division of Epidemiology and Public Health, Medical School, University of Newcastle upon Tyne.

Michael Hirst   Social Policy Research Unit, University of York.

PREFACE TO THE PAPERBACK EDITION

The research on which contributions to this book are based predates recent major reforms to both health and social care. Policy changes in the National Health Service, through *Caring for Patients* and to social services through the community care legislation, have introduced quasi-markets and the separation of the purchasers of services from the providers. These policy changes make quality of life measures even more important. Purchasers in both health and local authorities are required to assess needs of individuals and populations, a process which entails examination of the potential consequences of different interventions. Devising contracts for services requires providers to be more explicit both about the process of helping individuals and their families and the outcome of care on their quality of life. Contracts, audit and quality assurance, provide scope for the monitoring of the quality of services and their outcomes.

In the early stages of implementing these reforms there has been a concentration on the use of currently available but very limited data. Development of both health and social care services within the new policy framework will clearly require better measures of the quality of life. The contents of this book have therefore considerable relevance in the new policy climate.

Issues concerning the theoretical bases, statistical nature and application of quality of life measures are addressed in this volume from a number of social science perspectives. The question of whose quality of life, the cared-for, carer or family; the importance of individual autonomy; and the difficulties of monitoring quality of services are also considered. The problems that arise in using these measures for policy decisions, particularly in priority setting, are debated. All these issues retain their importance in the new quasi-markets.

It was possible to make only minor changes to the material from the original edition. However, while considerable research has been completed since the book has been published, most of the issues raised in this volume have not been resolved. The reissue of this volume therefore brings a welcome opportunity to reexamine the debates. We believe that the material from this book will continue to provide a stimulus to the examination of quality of life measurement at a time when its importance in the policy arena is more visible, and more important, than when it was first published.

Sally Baldwin
Christine Godfrey
Carol Propper

April 1993

ACKNOWLEDGEMENTS

The final form of this book owes much to the discussion held at the Institute for Research in the Social Sciences (IRISS) conference 'Quality of Life: perspectives and policies' held at the University of York, 11–12 November 1987. We are grateful to Professor Keith Hartley (Director, IRISS) for his encouragement and for the financial support provided by IRISS. We are also greatly indebted to Barbara Dodds and Dr Robert Walker for their invaluable help in organizing the conference. A large number of people contributed to the success of the conference. We gratefully acknowledge the contributions of contributors, chairs, and discussants not included in this collection: Mr Akehurst, Dr Ashmore, Mr Bone, Professor Bradshaw, Dr Dimitriou, Dr Gibbs, Professor Hutton, Dr Lavers, Dr Leonard, Dr Lowe, Professor Mulkay, Dr Normand, Dr Oldman, Dr Pinch, Professor Sawyer, Dr Twigg, and Professor Williams.

INTRODUCTION

SALLY BALDWIN, CHRISTINE GODFREY, and
CAROL PROPPER

Concern about the quality of life is by no means new, and such
concern is not, of course, the monopoly of social scientists. However,
recent developments in the fields of economics and social policy,
coupled with changes in the policy environment, have intensified
the interest of social scientists in particular aspects of quality of life.
Economic analysis of markets in which prices are absent, such as the
health and social services markets, has brought to the fore the
question of appropriate measures of output and outcome. To evaluate interventions in the field of acute health care, economists have
begun to develop quality of life measures. While not necessarily an
output measure, change in the quality of patients' lives is clearly one
outcome of an intervention in the market. In the field of social policy
the value of government intervention itself has come under scrutiny.
Liberal and libertarian critiques of state welfare have argued that
government intervention does not improve the quality of life of
recipients of welfare programmes and, indeed, ultimately damages
it. Such critiques have renewed interest in clarifying the objectives
and outcomes of government interventions and also in the question
of how exactly policy outcomes relate to the quality of life of those
receiving services.

Changes in the public sphere have also been important in
focusing attention on quality of life. In the last decade government
policy has increasingly been concerned with value for money. To
justify new or continued funding projects or programmes must be
shown, or appear to be, 'cost effective'. Social scientists have been
drawn into this process – both directly, as assessors of the cost-
effectiveness of policies, and indirectly, as the political climate has
shaped research priorities and research budgets. Clearly, measuring

1

cost-effectiveness requires not only the relatively straightforward task of quantifying inputs to a programme but also the more difficult task of evaluating its outcomes. Researchers have increasingly sought to assess policy in these terms, and have therefore had to tackle the difficult problems of identifying and measuring outputs and outcomes. As intermediate and final outputs have been disentangled change in quality of life has emerged as a critical component of outcome. The papers in this book demonstrate that the definition and measurement of quality of life is neither easy to resolve nor possible to ignore.

The papers presented here derive from a conference on the issue of quality of life held by the Institute for Research in the Social Sciences (IRISS) at the University of York on 11–12 November 1987. IRISS is the umbrella organization to which all those engaged in social science research at the University belong and the conference was the first in an annual series aiming to create a forum for researchers working on common topics. Participants came from different fields within the social sciences and the book reflects their different disciplinary backgrounds and interests. The issues addressed range from the philosophical question of what constitutes the good life to detailed studies of what constitutes a good quality of life for particular client groups; from technical discussion of the features of a quality of life measure to scrutiny of the difficult, and possibly controversial, implications of using such a measure as part of the resource allocation process.

It is clear from the papers presented in this book that the conference identified a number of key issues. It is also clear that these cross disciplinary boundaries. Interest in what constitutes the good life is not confined to philosophers; this issue must also be tackled by the researcher seeking to evaluate the development of new arrangements for fostering, or the effects of seeking to support people with mental handicaps in community settings. Nor is the question of measurement the sole preserve of the technically orientated, since the measures developed may determine the allocation of scarce resources and hence who receives, or does not receive, health care, social services, or social security benefits. At the extreme such measures could be used as part of the process which defines some individuals in society as deserving and others as undeserving, perhaps ultimately of who should live, and who will therefore die. That this process may occur is not a reason for halting the development of such outcome measures. It is, rather, an even stronger reason for clarifying the issues involved in their development and opening up the process to critical scrutiny.

The critical issues identified in the conference and addressed in this volume revolve around the search for, development, use, and implications of a measure (or set of measures) of quality of life. The researchers who have contributed to the book have in common the recognition that quality of life is a multidimensional concept; however, they display considerable divergence in approach. Their interest is motivated by different concerns and requirements. The contributors bring perspectives from a number of disciplinary backgrounds and examine these issues in varying contexts. This divergence is, we feel, a strength. Academic research is typically carried out and disseminated within narrow disciplinary boundaries; the similarities and contrasts between different approaches to common questions are rarely explored. The multidisciplinary nature of this book has enabled us to engage in such an exploration.

The collection begins with an examination of the philosophical basis of the concept of quality of life. It is obvious from the three papers in this section that there are a number of possible starting points, each of which will yield a different type of measure and each of which embodies an explicit or implicit set of assumptions about the important dimensions of quality of life. Megone (Chapter Two) puts forward the case for a single measure which remains unchanged through time and societies, based on our essential nature as rational beings. In contrast, Hodge (Chapter Three) argues that any measure must be viewed as the product of the society in which it is used and, further, that different philosophical schools of thought imply different measures and uses for such measures. She argues that no single measure is suitable for all policy evaluation; that, if such a measure is used, the researcher has to some extent already determined the kind of questions that can be asked and therefore the kind of answers that can be produced. On the other hand, Culyer (Chapter One) argues that the economist's traditional tool, the utilitarian framework, can be extended to encompass many of the relevant aspects of quality of life. He argues that this may be achieved by replacing the standard arguments of the utility function, namely *commodities*, with *characteristics*. Interestingly, it is Hodge's theme which is echoed later in the book by Shiell *et al.* (Chapter Seven) in discussing the use of economic frameworks to evaluate different ways of providing care for people who are mentally handicapped.

Part Two of the book focuses on the development of a measure of quality of life that can be used in policy evaluation. A central issue is whether it is possible, useful, or appropriate to develop a single measure. The single measure need not be based on one dimension. Different dimensions of life quality may be combined to produce a single measure. It is recognized that a single measure has considerable advantages, not least that it permits comparison with other single measures, such as money, and so can easily be used in cost-benefit analyses. It also allows comparisons to be made across individuals and between programmes with different objectives and which affect different client groups. A single measure is clearly attractive to policy makers. Some of the methodological issues in the development of such a measure are examined in depth in the paper by Kind (Chapter Four).

Unitary measures, however, have been subject to criticism both on technical and on broader philosophical and political grounds. The technical process of measure development may be considered to have three stages. The choice of dimensions constitutes the first stage. The second involves the valuation of the different dimensions, which may be extremely difficult to quantify – for example, aspects of quality of life such as pain or distress. The third stage involves the combination of the different dimensions by some scaling process. The selection of dimensions, the seeking of valuations, and the combination of dimensions have all proved to be controversial.

Loomes and McKenzie (Chapter Six) scrutinize one measure of quality of life which has been developed within the context of health care provision, and enables the user to rank the benefits of different treatments on a single scale. This measure is the Quality Adjusted Life Year (QALY). They argue that this measure may produce inconsistent results when used to select between different forms of treatment for the same individual, and also when choices must be made between alternative ways of allocating limited resources among diverse health care activities.

Hirst (Chapter Five) argues that quality of life is inherently multi-dimensional and that measures of the concept should therefore retain this multidimensional nature. He presents a methodology for describing quality of life which does not involve any loss of information. He illustrates its use within the context of analysis of disability, but stresses that the technique is applicable to a wide range of situations.

Hodge's discussion of the potential uses and abuses of a single measure provides a reminder of some political and philosophical problems of single measures. So, from different perspectives, do all the papers in Part Three. In this section, researchers from a number of disciplines draw on empirical research to examine aspects of quality of life in particular settings, institutional and non-institutional. Shiell *et al.* (Chapter Seven) argue that the QALY measure, developed in the context of allocation of acute medical care, is not helpful in considering improvements in the outcome for those with mental handicaps. Parker (Chapter Eight) brings to our attention the danger, perhaps fostered by use of a single measure, of focusing only on the individuals directly affected by illness or disability. Drawing on research into the effects on spouses of caring for partners who have become disabled, she stresses that misfortune of this sort affects not only the quality of life of the disabled person, but also that of the carer. In addition, the nature of the interaction between carer and cared-for is itself an important component of the quality of life of each individual. A measure that examines only the quality of life of the person who is sick or disabled would omit these important considerations. The contributions of Downes (Chapter Ten), Corden (Chapter Eleven), and Baldwin and Gerard (Chapter Nine) signal the diversity of factors which may influence quality of life. Downes suggests that autonomy may be an important factor in determining the success of foster placements for 'difficult' adolescents. Corden suggests that choice may be a key factor for the quality of life of elderly people in residential care. Baldwin and Gerard review the aspects of mental handicap in a child that can affect the quality of life both of the child and of its family. In addition to illustrating the wide range of factors which can determine the quality of life these papers also indicate that, in the field of social care, research is at an early stage in its contribution to both measurement and evaluation. In many situations we are only at the beginning of the process: at the stage where we can begin to identify relevant dimensions; in a position only to reject some and perhaps concentrate on others. Identification, rather than measurement, is often the main aim of the researcher.

Hutton (Chapter Twelve) takes rather a different route. She seeks to examine the extent to which quality of life is associated with income. To do this, she uses micro-data to examine the association between income and other goods which have been taken as indicators of quality of life, exploring whether there is a point below which the quality of life of people with low incomes diverges sharply from that enjoyed by the rest of society.

The papers in the fourth and final section all address the interface between quality of life and government policy. The common theme across all three papers is the inter-relationship between individuals and society when resources are constrained. Gudex (Chapter Fourteen) explores the implications of using QALY measures to allocate resources between different health care uses. Godfrey and Powell (Chapter Thirteen) discuss the appropriateness of using economic models to analyse government interventions in order to stop individuals from pursuing personal self-interest in the consumption of hazardous goods. Finally, Eastwood and Maynard (Chapter Fifteen) discuss the treatment of Acquired Immune Deficiency (AIDS), attempt to assess the cost per QALY of treating people with AIDS, and examine the ethical problems that are raised by the high cost of treatment. From the research in this section it is clear that measuring quality of life does not resolve issues of resource allocation. If anything, the potential conflicts and ethical issues implicit in seeking to allocate resources on the basis of an explicit quality of life measure emerge more strongly when the implications of decisions are clarified.

The chapters in this volume provide ideas about and research tools with which to examine quality of life. The collection highlights the benefits of collaborative cross-disciplinary research. It is clear that researchers are being impelled to confront similar issues from within traditionally separate disciplines. It is also clear that we can learn by making links between these research endeavours – within and between applied researchers, those engaged in theoretical debate, and those engaged in policy analysis. Manifestly there remain many issues to be explored, and there are real differences and disagreements in the way similar problems are conceptualized and addressed within the social sciences. This book is intended as a stimulus towards the further examination of quality of life and perhaps also to the resolution of some of the problems and conflicts identified here.

Part One

CONCEPTUAL
FRAMEWORKS

COMMODITIES, CHARACTERISTICS OF COMMODITIES, CHARACTERISTICS OF PEOPLE, UTILITIES, AND THE QUALITY OF LIFE

A. J. CULYER[1]

This paper tries to set research into the quality of life – especially in the sub-territory of QALY research and health status measurement – into a wider context that taxonomizes concerns of both researchers and their customers, and of researchers coming from different disciplinary backgrounds, according to thing- and people-orientation. Within this framework I shall try to show that the limitations of welfarism and utilitarianism as normative frameworks for discussing quality of life, though profound, paradoxically emphasize the importance of utility theory. I shall also try to show that there are many unresolved ethical questions. One is whether quality of life is to be seen as an absolute or relative idea. Another is whether taking account of distributional aspects of the quality of life or standards of living is done best by looking at outcome distribution, the commodity distribution, or by applying individual *a priori* weights to relevant characteristics of people. Because social scientists do not share common meanings even when they use common words (like welfare, utility, utilitarian, and relative) I have tried to make clear my own meanings and hope that any residual ambiguity will not materially get in the reader's way.

I want to begin by making some distinctions based on ideas developed by Sen (1982:30). The key idea is to distinguish between categories describing *things* and their characteristics on the one hand, and *people* and theirs on the other. The distinction between the two is not advanced as any kind of fundamental Cartesian

9

dualism but rather as a heuristic device that usefully introduces a thought-provoking symmetry in the principal approaches to quality of life that are found in the literature. Even as a heuristic device, as will be seen later, it has some limitations. For the moment, however, it serves.

On the left hand side of Figure 1.1 is 'the universe of things'. This consists of commodities, that is, goods and services in the everyday sense, whose demand and supply, and whose growth, have been a traditional focus of economists' attention and whose personal distribution has been a traditional focus of all social scientists having an interest in distributive justice. These commodities have characteristics. It also happens that these characteristics are a way in which we often describe the quality of goods. It is self-evident that the quality of *commodities* is not at all, however, the same thing as the quality of *life*.

In explaining aspects of consumer behaviour some economists (notably Lancaster 1971) have reinterpreted traditional demand theory (for commodities) as a demand for *characteristics* (of commodities). This has been done by supposing that rational utility maximizers derive utility not so much from goods and services *per se*, as in the traditional approach, as from the characteristics of goods. In terms of the first example in Figure 1.1: the demand for steaks is to be explored in terms of the demand for the characteristics of steaks (juiciness, etc.). Similarly, the welfare (or quality of life) of individuals is to be explored in terms of the utility of characteristics such as these.

Both traditional welfare economics and the 'characteristics' approach proceed to utility (provisionally taken as synonymous with happiness or pleasure – more on this anon) directly without the intervening category 'characteristics of people' (we had better avoid the seemingly eugenic term 'quality of people'). It is in this way that quality of life is usually defined: either directly in terms of the 'welfare' that is got from goods, or indirectly in terms of the 'welfare' that is got from the characteristics of goods.

The intervening category consists of *non-utility* information about people. This may relate back (in a causal way) to the consumption of either commodities or the characteristics of commodities. It may also simply relate to inherent characteristics of people – for example, their genetic endowment of health, their relative deprivation independent of the absolute consumption of commodities or the

10

Figure 1.1 Relationship between commodities, characteristics, and utilities

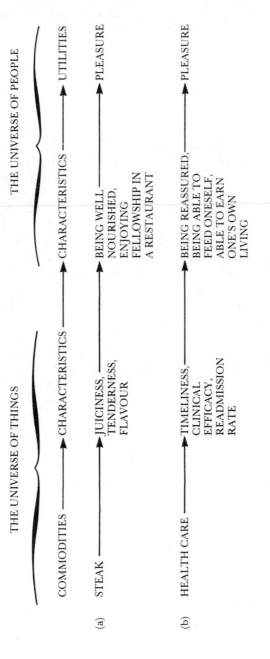

characteristics of commodities, their moral 'worth' and 'deserving-ness'. It may, further, relate to the character of relationships between people such as the quality of friendships, community support for the individual when in need, social isolation, or changes in them, such as becoming (as distinct from being) divorced.

These non-utility bits of information about people do not usually form a part of the conventional measurement of standards of living (at least in the work of economists) though the 'social indicators movement' has consistently taken a non-utility focus. The conventional approach was, on the contrary, what one may call *welfarist* (Sen 1979). Welfarism holds that the standard of living, quality of life, efficiency of social arrangements, even the justice of distributions and redistributions, are all to be judged or evaluated in terms of the utilities of the individuals concerned. I use the term *utilitarianism* to denote a specific form of welfarism using the additional ethical principle that the total utility, or average utility, ought to be maximized. The Paretian method of welfare economics is also welfarist though it is not utilitarian in the rather restrictive sense in which I am using the term.

The explicit introduction of *characteristics of people* opens up an alternative or supplementary, non-utility, view of the quality of life, defined in terms of these characteristics. As in the first example in Figure 1.1, the characteristics may be related to levels of nourishment, fellowship at meal times, and the like. This approach seems to be characteristic of, for example, Townsend's (1979) concept of poverty (though that is rather heavily commodities-focused). It is also characteristic of the health measurement movement, QALYs, health indices, and all that. The categorization in Figure 1.1 is also one into which at least one tradition in the discussion of 'need' fits (e.g. Culyer 1976). If the characteristics of people are a way of describing deprivation, desired states, or significant changes in people's characteristics, then commodities and characteristics of commodities are what is often needed to remove the deprivation or to move towards the desired state, or to help people cope with change. They are the necessary means to a desired end. To compare the *ill-health* of different individuals or groups is not the same as to compare the *health care* they have received (they could receive the same amounts and still be unhealthy, or different amounts and be equally healthy). Nor is it the same as their *pleasure* (a sick optimist may have far more pleasure from life than a well grumbler). In

12

short, a focus on characteristics of people is not the same as a focus on commodities, characteristics of commodities, or utilities and it has some distinct advantages over these other approaches.

WHY CHARACTERISTICS, NOT UTILITIES?

One set of reasons for paying more attention to characteristics than utilities has been given by Williams:

> The characteristic approach of economists to the valuation of social goods is to try to find some private good which is systematically related to it, and by measuring the values people place on the latter, make some inferences about the implicit (upper or lower bounds of) values they place on the former. . . . On occasions, however, social policy confronts problems where the community has explicitly rejected one or another of the basic assumptions on which this approach rests. Among these basic assumptions, two are especially important: (1) people are the best (or even sometimes the sole) judges of their own welfare; and (2) the preferences of different individuals are to be weighted according to the prevailing distribution of income and wealth. In some areas of social policy (e.g. mental illness and physical handicap), the first assumption is challenged, and over a much wider range of social concerns the second one is considered ethically unacceptable as the basis for public policy valuations.
>
> (Williams 1977:282)

This paper – while not dissenting from Williams' arguments – makes a rather more general argument for the 'characteristics of people' approach: more general in the sense that it will encompass both efficiency and distributional types of concern and more general also in the sense that it transcends traditional utilitarianism.

The odd idea has grown up (even amongst non-economists) that welfarism is the economist's *only* way of approaching these questions. For example, in discussing Williams (1985) on QALYs, Smith (1987:1135) stated: 'A cost-effectiveness approach to the allo-cation of health resources presupposes a simple utilitarian or Benthamite concept of justice.' Fortunately that is not so – and it is fortunate not only because the sort of things that concern Smith (the variance in rather than the unweighted sum total of 'health') are themselves as exclusive as welfarism. It is just not true that the QALY/CEA approach commits us to 'simple' welfarist concepts (for example, less 'simple' are maximin notions or a specially weighted sum of utilities). More important is that the QALY/CEA approach need not be utilitarian at all. For, although the QALY/CEA approach *can* focus on the fourth column in Figure 1.1 (utility), it can also focus on the third column: characteristics of people. To focus here is *not* to focus on utility.

Suppose that there were two individuals whose claims on resources were being assessed. One is a perfect pleasure machine who gets ten times more pleasure out of a given income than the other, a chronic arthritic. 'Simple' utilitarianism will take no cognizance of this fact, focusing on the *marginal* utility of each. If the arthritic had a lower marginal utility of income than the pleasure machine, simple utilitarianism would have us take income from him or her and transfer it to the pleasure machine, because the utility loss to the low marginal utility person will be smaller than the utility gain to the high marginal utility person, and arthritis is an irrelevance – unless suffering from it affects the utility of income (at the margin). Utilitarianism may even have us do that if the pleasure machine were already richer (in income) than the arthritic, provided of course that the machine's utility gain still exceeded the poor and arthritic person's utility loss.

Now that seems out of tune with what we intuit to be the right thing to do. Suppose, then, one focused on total utilities instead of the marginal. (Can one take this to be a slightly less 'simple' utilitarianism?) Suppose one wanted to equalize each person's utility as much as possible given their initial combined incomes. If the arthritic had lower utility than the pleasure machine all would be well, or at least, if not *all*, the redistribution would go in the right direction (just as it would had the arthritic had a higher marginal utility of income under 'simple' utilitarianism). But now suppose that is not the case. The arthritic, despite the pain and incapacity, has an invariably sunny disposition while the pleasure machine, though efficient at manufacturing pleasure out of income, is of a melancholic cast, a Calvinist convinced of not being among the chosen. Now, even if the arthritic has the higher marginal utility of income, we shall no longer even judge that state to be deprived (in terms of total utility or pleasure). Once again, something seems to have gone wrong. Intuition tells us that the arthritic is in some sort

14

of need, does need help, is deserving of our sympathy.

What may be going wrong is that the utilitarian approach, like all welfarist approaches, rejects all non-utility information about people as being irrelevant in judgements about efficiency and justice. This is why I said earlier that it was 'fortunate' that the QALY/CEA approach to decision making is not dependent on welfarist concepts, for it is its ability to exploit other descriptive characteristics of people (like whether they are crippled from arthritis) that makes it decisively non-welfarist.

Sen (1980) has developed the notion of 'basic capabilities'. These refer to one's *capability of functioning*: what one can do — getting around, looking after oneself (and others), earning a living, having discussions about the quality of life, and so on. If you think of 'standard of living' or 'quality of life' in terms of capabilities of functioning then you can immediately see that one may be rich (have lots of commodities) but have a low standard of living. One may be deliriously happy (have lots of utility) but have a low standard of living. Sen's notion of capabilities thus shares with my 'characteristics of people' the idea that *utility* focuses too much on mental and emotional responses to commodities and characteristics of commodities and not enough on what they enable you to do.

The notion of basic capabilities has lots of attractions. One is that it seems to provide what is missing in welfarism. Another is its evident culture-contingency. (Some may dub it 'relative' but I prefer to use this adjective in a more restrictive sense.) Yet another is the (again evident) way in which the notion encourages practical people to think explicitly about the capabilities that are to be reckoned relevant, how they are to be weighted, and so on. Yet we should be cautious before committing ourselves to the 'basic capabilities' approach. For one thing, we need to give a lot more thought to the meaning and significance of 'basic'. Indeed, it may be prudent to use the more general notion of 'characteristics of people' rather than 'basic capabilities' precisely because it does not involve the prior exclusion of some characteristics (whatever they may be) that the criterion of 'basic' (whatever it may be) clearly does.

Another reason for caution is that it does not seem that *only* capabilities enter the notion of 'standard of living' or 'quality of life'. There are other attributes that we may want to add in that are still not commodities, characteristics of commodities, or utility, but neither are they capabilities. If our arthritic is in *pain*, that is a factor

15

to take account of in assessing the quality of life. If the arthritic is bereft of friends, that too should be taken into account. So is whether or not a person is stigmatized (even if the stigma does not deprive a person of commodities). 'Characteristics' seems to me to be altogether a more open category and one capable of exciting the imagination out of conventional and tram-lined ways of thinking about quality of life.

There is a further reason for judging the characteristics approach a good one: it enables a more effective cross-disciplinary dialogue. For example, the characteristics approach to social deprivation is extremely sympathetic to Townsend's approach to poverty measurement and, indeed, provides a systematic theoretical underpinning for it (but see Townsend 1985). More importantly, the characteristics approach, even in its 'basic capabilities' version, like all good theoretical underpinnings, has the ability to clarify and surprise. It has that quality so nicely termed 'Aha-ness' by Blaug (1980:6).

UTILITY WITHOUT UTILITARIANISM

One should caution against a too complete rejection of utilitarianism. Indeed, there is one respect in which utilitarianism has a great deal to offer even those committing themselves to a 'characteristics of people' approach.

Etzioni (1986) has identified three main variations in economists' use of the concept of utility. First is the original concept, that of the pleasure of the self, which has been used in this paper so far. This concept provides the human psychology of neo-classical economics and underlies the ethics of welfarism.

The second is an expanded version of the first encompassing the satisfactions a person gains both from his own consumption of goods (or characteristics of goods) and from that of others. This is utility interdependence, a species of externality, that is increasingly used (though still not widely) by economists working on topics in social policy, and that has given rise to economic interpretations of altruism and caring (e.g. Culyer 1983).

The third is the use of the term 'utility' as a formal attribute, having no substantive attributes: a means merely of ranking preferences or choices. As Alchian put it:

For analytical convenience it is customary to postulate that an

16

individual seeks to maximize something subject to some constraints. The thing – or numerical measure of the 'thing' – which he seeks to maximize is called 'utility'. Whether or not utility is some kind of glow or warmth, or happiness, is here irrelevant; all that counts is that we can assign numbers to entities or conditions which a person can strive to realize. Then we say the individual seeks to maximize some function of those numbers. Unfortunately, the term 'utility' has by now acquired so many connotations, that it is difficult to realize that for the present purposes *utility has no more meaning than this*.

(Alchian 1953:73; italics added)

Etzioni condemns all three forms of what he calls the 'mono-utility paradigm' on the grounds that they omit too much that is relevant (echoes on the behavioural front of Sen on the ethical) and in particular he heaps scorn on the poverty of the third use as a motivational basis for behaviour (animal or human).

This condemnation, no matter how right on the grounds of making a satisfactory theory of human behaviour, seems too total. In particular, I want to argue (not for the first time, see Culyer 1983) that the third usage of the concept of 'utility' is important even for those espousing the 'characteristics of people' approach to measuring the quality of life. Its importance is twofold: in the first place, by its extensive exploration of 'measurement' the literature has clarified important meanings (e.g. ordinal, interval, and ratio scales), identified false interpretations (e.g. the non-uniqueness of elasticity measures of dependent variables measured on linear scales), and yielded up experimental techniques like the rating scale, the standard gamble, and the time trade-off method for the empirical study of the values that people have (and the differences that exist between them) (Torrance 1986). In the second place, this genre of the literature very precisely pinpoints the need for value-judgements: not merely about the selection of the characteristics to be included in an assessment of the quality of life, but also about the selection of the selectors; not only about the scaling of characteristics as 'better' or 'worse', but also about the ways in which characteristics should be traded-off; not only about overall weighted measures of the quality of life of one kind (for example, health) but how that compares (and interacts) with other aspects of the quality of life (for example, education). It is notable that any systematic consideration of these aspects of the inherent value-content of quality of life measurement is often wholly absent from discussions of quality of life that are not informed by utility theory (e.g. Townsend 1979).

These advantages of utility theory are most to the fore when one is dealing with multi-attribute notions of poverty, quality of life, health, and so on. As a practical matter it frequently happens that one is comparing individuals (or the same individual over time) for whom some attributes worsen and others improve. This is a good example of a way in which an aggregation process, instead of 'destroying' information, can actually create it: specifically creating information about the severity (etc.) with which various attributes (whether they be commodities or characteristics) are regarded and the degree to which improvement in one (or more) may be regarded as compensating for worsening in others. Unless the researcher is prepared with a method for dealing with these issues there will be little alternative than to have recourse to arbitrary (usually personal) value judgements which may be proper for parents, or even social workers, but are scarcely appropriate for social scientists.

Utility, therefore, remains a core concept, and the lessons learned about its measurability, its measurement, and the necessarily value-laden steps needed to put substantive content into the abstract notion are essential lessons, even if you are not a welfarist. You still need utility theory even if you aren't a utilitarian!

There is an aspect of these claims of 'clarifying' and 'pinpointing' (which many of us are wont to make) that is extraordinarily perplexing and not a little disturbing. Despite the explicitness of the non-utilitarian use of utility theory and the fact that the QALY approach to quality of life in health matters has repeatedly – and again explicitly – drawn attention to its value-judgemental content, readers whom one would take as normally sophisticated frequently interpret the approach in grotesquely perverse ways. Smith, for example, believes that the old and the very sick are necessarily discriminated against by the QALY approach and that a quantitative algorithm obscures the fact that arbitrary assessments of value are being made (Smith 1987). The truth is, however, that the QALY approach can be made to 'discriminate' (if that's the word you want to use) against or in favour of whomsoever one pleases while it has nothing at all to say about how the assessments of value *ought* to be made (let alone that they should be arbitrary). It has, by contrast, many suggestions about how they *can*, as a matter of fact, be made.

18

QUALITY OF LIFE: RELATIVE OR ABSOLUTE

One of the features of 'characteristics of people' to which I earlier drew attention is that relationships and positional aspects may be included amongst them. Sen has used the distinctions of Figure 1.1 in order to comment on the literature of relative deprivation (a literature whose contribution to the discussion of poverty he regards as valuable). In particular, he argues the subtle point that *absolute* deprivation in capabilities (but I shall continue to use the more inclusive 'characteristics of people') relates to *relative* deprivation in terms of commodities.

This adds a useful insight into the meaning of poverty. The argument is that poverty is an absolute notion to do with the characteristics of people rather than a purely relative one (in the sense of a ratio rather than context-dependent), though it remains relative (again in the ratio sense) in the universe of commodities. For example, the absolute element in poverty relates, let us suppose, to a further notion of being a member of the community. Being relatively deprived of particular commodities denies one this full membership. The absolute element is not fixed. It takes different things in different times and different places to enable each person to be identified as a member of the group. You can even conceive of 'degrees of membership' (e.g. first- and second-class citizenship). But, for all that, the basic notion is an absolute one and is to do with characteristics of people. The relativist notion depends upon your access, possession, ownership, entitlement, and so on, to and of commodities relative to others. That is why poverty in Britain is different, and differently seen, from poverty in Bangladesh. That is why, in today's Britain, it is important (following Townsend 1979) not to be deprived of holidays, TV sets, and Christmas presents. But, if you are relatively deprived of these things, and in Britain today, you are absolutely poor.

The distinction may seem elusive. For a good example of how it can elude some subtle minds, see Townsend (1985) and Sen's reply (1985). It is rather like the notion of positional goods discussed by Hirsch (1977): if you want to enjoy the absolute advantage of sunbathing on an uncrowded beach, your ability to do so may well depend on your relative knowledge of the various available beaches compared with the knowledge of others. A differential advantage in information gives you an absolute advantage in enjoying the beach.

19

Sen gives an example from Adam Smith: 'the Greeks and Romans lived . . . very comfortably though they had no linen, [but] in the present time, through the greater part of Europe, a creditable day-labourer would be ashamed to appear in public without a linen shirt' (1983:161). To avoid shame in different contexts and times may require different bundles of commodities and the bundles required (and the resources to acquire them) will often be defined relative to the bundles (and resources) of other people. But the avoidance of the shame is absolute not relative. It is not a question of being more or less ashamed, or even of having equal shame, but of avoiding shame altogether: absolutely.

If one were to take another negative aspect of the quality of life, unemployment, cannot a similar argument be mounted? For example, even if the benefits in cash and kind available to the unemployed were sufficient to protect them from poverty, unemployment remains an evil (and not merely an inefficient use – or, rather, non-use – of resources). This is because unemployment is doubly stigmatizing: one is stigmatized in one's own eyes as a failure and one is stigmatized publicly in the eyes of others. To avoid stigma it is necessary in our culture for people of particular ages, sexes, and physical and mental abilities to have employment. Stigma is absolute; the avoidance of stigma is absolute. This is perfectly consistent with the possibility of stigma being *scalable* (*viz* measurable) in terms of more or less, worse or better. Stigma, of whatever degree, is the state you are in – but whether you are in it depends on your employment status *relative to* others. *That* status is positional. If no one works, no one is stigmatized. Among some South American tribes the skin disease, pinto, was so prevalent that those single men *not* suffering from it were regarded as pathological and excluded from marriage (Ackerknecht 1947). (For other medical and sociological examples of relativist-absolutist interractions in health see Culyer 1978:96ff.)

But we are running into difficulties with Figure 1.1, for the descriptor 'unemployed' is not descriptive of commodities but of people. What we have is some absolute characteristics of people being determined by some other relative characteristics of people. The framework seems to need enlargement to meet this important dimension of quality of life. That is a task I am not going to tackle here.

Relativism seems less important in health than in some other aspects of the quality of life, and this despite the well-known culture dependency of attitudes to pain, disability, and disease. In general, it seems that it is not the case that absolute notions of health (no matter how variable or culture-bound they may be) are dependent upon positional information about someone's relative access to care, their relative limitation of functional activity, and so on. Relativism does not usually play any major role in how we conceptualize or measure 'health'. The arrows in Figure 1.1 still convey the right sense of movement from left to right. Instead, however, of having (relative) lack of goods → (absolute) poverty, we have (absolute) lack of health care, (absolute) presence of harmful pathogens, (absolute) prevalence of risky lifestyles → (absolute) poor health.

The same can probably not be said for quality of life itself. It is not very controversial to suggest that quality of life is to do with shared views about how one ought to be able to live. It is at least in part to do with the absolute characteristics of people. It is by derivation to do with commodities or their characteristics. But just as the general view about what a minimum 'decent' (absolute) quality of life or standard of living is can vary over time and place, so can the relationship which the quality of life has to the commodities contributing to it.

What is more difficult to determine is whether the instrumental role of commodities, or characteristics of commodities, is relative or absolute. In part it is clearly relative: the 'keeping up with Joneses' effect. But it is also no less clearly absolute: I believe the quality of my life rises when I have more of particular commodities independently of whether I have *relatively* more. It is *not* the same to me whether I have £1,000 more commodities per year or everyone else has £1,000 each less.

My tentative conclusion is thus that in the meaning of 'poverty', relativity in commodities is very important. In the meaning of 'health', relativity in commodities hardly matters at all. In the meaning of 'quality of life' relativity and absoluteness in commodities both matter. In all three cases, poverty, health, and quality of life, the descriptive condition itself as a bundle of characteristics of people is, however, absolute.

But in thus relegating relativism to a backseat in health, I do not want to be taken as automatically relegating *inequality* also to a backseat. Indeed, the question 'inequality of what?' in health policy is an issue that arises partly out of the taxonomy of Figure 1.1, and the instrumental link between commodities, their characteristics, and the characteristics of people.

HEALTH CARE: EQUALITY OF WHAT?

There is a phrase in Smith's (1987) paper which is notable for having been picked up by none of his critics (Williams 1987; Evans 1987; Drummond 1987): 'a traditional clinical view would favour policies designed to allocate resources to those most in need of them with the general objective of reducing health variance' (Smith 1987:1135). It is not, perhaps, plausible to suppose that this really has been a traditional clinical view (it probably all depends upon the tradition!) but that should not distract our attention from the key idea that a distributional rather than a maximizing/optimizing objective should command centre-stage.

One way of sharpening up perceptions about distributions is to look at some examples and ask ourselves what we think about them. Imagine that we have some non-controversial measure of health as a characteristic of people like QALYs measured on a ratio scale(!), a limited budget denominated in commodity units of resource, and a knowledge of the technology for transforming existing health states into better ones, as well as of the natural history of the diseases in question (so that we also know, for example, what happens if we do nothing).

With those immodest requirements taken for granted, consider Table 1.1A. This shows three distributions: the first column shows a starting distribution of average health status per person across disease classifications, geographical regions or whatever (a, b, c, d). The second shows a distribution of twenty commodity units of resources (a stock taken as given for the purposes of the exercise) which, in Table 1.1A, is optimally distributed so as to maximize its impact on health. The resultant distribution of health is shown in the third column: given the starting point, commodities, prevailing technology, etc., the maximum final sum of health statuses is 250. The total product of the twenty resource units is, incidentally, 120 (the difference between the final sum and what the sum would have been had no commodity-resources been applied) not twenty (the difference between the final and the initial totals). This you can infer from the information provided in Table 1.1D, which shows the marginal increases in health status from applying commodity-

22

resources in five unit increments. Table 1.1A is thus showing what I take to be the 'simple utilitarian' view that so distressed Smith.

Table 1.1B has the same initial distribution of health but a different distribution of the twenty units of commodities. Here they have been so applied as to reduce the variance in health to zero. The result is not only to reduce overall health status relative to the optimal (utilitarian) distribution – as must necessarily be the case by virtue of that distribution's optimality – but also to reduce average health in the community as a whole. I rather doubt whether the 'traditional clinical view' values reductions in variance *that much*. I have

Table 1.1 Exemplary distributions of health, health care resources, and marginal products

A. Health maximization

(a)	100	————————	(5) ————————▶	100
(b)	80	————————	(10) ————————▶	100
(c)	40	————————	(5) ————————▶	50
(d)	10	————————	(0) ————————▶	0
	230		20	250

B. Health equalization

(a)	100	————————	(0) ————————▶	50
(b)	80	————————	(0) ————————▶	50
(c)	40	————————	(5) ————————▶	50
(d)	10	————————	(15) ————————▶	50
	230		20	200

C. Commodities equalization

(a)	100	————————	(5) ————————▶	100
(b)	80	————————	(5) ————————▶	70
(c)	40	————————	(5) ————————▶	50
(d)	10	————————	(5) ————————▶	10
	230		20	230

D. Marginal products of commodities

	Effect of doing nothing	Increasing resources from 0 to 5	Increasing resources from 5 to 10	Increasing resources from 10 to 15
(a)	−50	50	< 30	< 10
(b)	−30	20	30	< 10
(c)	−10	20	< 30	< 10
(d)	−10	10	30	10

made the numbers pose the question dramatically of course: but what *is* the acceptable price that one should pay for greater equality?

Table 1.1C again has the same starting distribution but aims for equality of *commodity* distribution rather than equality of the final health distribution. (Imagine, if you like, that each of the groups a, b, c, and d has equal numbers of people in it so that the commodity equality is commodity equality per head.) As it happens, this produces an outcome that is no worse in total than the initial total and is quite close to the total with the efficient commodity allocation. This feature has been deliberately built into the example in order to highlight what I conjecture may be the real concern of those who emphasize resource equality, namely that it approximates the optimal solution by concentrating more commodities on deprived groups for whom the marginal product of health services is relatively high. The equal resource distribution also lowers the variance of the final health distribution compared with the distribution associated with the optimal commodity deployment, though this is incidental for those whose ethical focus is on commodity equality alone. But, if it is true that 'commodity equalizers' are really covert outcome maximizers, their egalitarianism is entirely instrumental, justified because it is a useful rule of thumb rather than because it is inherently to be desired or is inherently ethical (Culyer 1988). When mere equality is not 'enough', such people will often advocate 'positive discrimination', thereby clearly proclaiming the (imperfect) instrumentality of commodity equalization. Instrumental egalitarianism seems worth differentiating from end-state egalitarianism. The reasoning in support of each is quite different and one certainly does not imply the other.

In considering the trade-off between efficiency and the equality of the final distribution it is interesting to ask whether the fact that one is dealing with 'health' makes any difference from when one is dealing with, say, 'income'. In both cases some gain and others lose as one moves from an equal to an efficient distribution, or vice versa. In both cases the efficient distribution has a larger total than the equal one. But does it make a difference that in the one case one is dealing with purchasing power and in the other with 'life'? Suppose, for example, that the health measure is 'lives saved' and that we make the value judgement that every life is of equal value whatever its length and quality and regardless of the intrinsic merits of the individuals in question. (I am not *advocating* these judgements.) In that case equality actually involves the sacrifice – the 'unnecessary' sacrifice in the sense that with the resources available the sacrifice could have been avoided – of people. Human sacrifices. Does that not matter? What further differences would be made if you disallowed the judgements that I just claimed not to be advocating? Suppose the numbers represented 'life years' – so that the sacrifice was not of entire lifetimes, but only parts of lifetimes? Or suppose they were QALYs, so the sacrifice was of the lowest quality life-years?

I do not know how others will answer these questions but I strongly suspect that, in order to answer them, one would want to adduce not only non-utility information but also non-health information, just as in discussing efficiency and social justice more generally there is a good case for seeking out non-utility information. The sort of information is familiar and it is to do with still other characteristics of people: age (do we not feel impelled to cherish the life-years of the very young and the very old?), desert (do we not feel differently about the person whose poor health is the result of their own reckless behaviour from the way we feel about the person who is prudent?), do we not have a special attitude to those in important social positions, and so on. And now suppose that you have *those* weights right. Indeed, suppose they are embodied in the numbers in the first column of Table 1.1. Is there any distributional concern left that has not been embodied? If not, the maximizers have the day (though not the 'simple utilitarians'). If so, then we are perhaps at the heart of what it is that the egalitarians fear most from the maximizers. But what it can be I cannot discern! And what relation it may have to the quality of life I cannot fathom.

END-PIECE

I hope to have given you some *prima facie* grounds for questioning some of the common approaches to the quality of life – especially those dubbed 'welfarist' and some prima facie *good* reasons for pursuing an alternative based on characteristics of people. I have argued that quantification of some sort is inescapable and that utility theory has some cautionary as well as practical lessons to teach in this regard (especially for those who fear or are sceptical about quantification). I have also suggested that the proposed way of looking at things has the potential for radically altering the ways in which we think and talk about distributive justice. For some this is not news. QALY researchers in particular have been using the characteristics of people approach and utility theory without utilitarianism for at least a decade. I have tried to show that this research programme can be seen as having its intellectual roots in a theory of the quality of life that encompasses, but is much more general than, the particular ethical apparatuses traditionally used by economists and other social scientists, and that this theory opens up a wide range of interesting and important questions both of principle and practice.

NOTE

1 I have benefited from correspondence with Amitai Etzioni, Michael Mulkay, Amartya Sen, Alwyn Smith, and Peter Townsend, from discussions at the conference, and I am also grateful for the comments of the editors.

REFERENCES

Ackerknecht, E. W. (1947) 'The role of medical history in medical education', *Bulletin of the History of Medicine* 21.
Alchian, A. A. (1953) 'The meaning of utility measurement', *American Economic Review* 26–50. Reprinted in W. Breit and H.M. Hochman (eds) *Readings in Microeconomics*, New York: Holt, Rinehart, & Winston. (This is the version from which the quotation in the text comes.)
Blaug, M. (1980) *The Methodology of Economics*, Cambridge: Cambridge University Press.
Culyer, A. J. (1976) *Need and the National Health Service: Economics and Social Choice*, London: Martin Robertson.
Culyer, A. J. (1983) 'Economics without economic man?', *Social Policy and Administration* 17:188–203.
Culyer, A. J. (1988) *Measuring Health: Lessons for Ontario*, Toronto: University of Toronto Press.
Culyer, A. J. (1988) 'Inequality of health services is, in general, desirable', in D. Green (ed.) *Acceptable Inequalities*, London: Institute of Economic Affairs.
Drummond, M. F. (1987) letter to *The Lancet*, i:1372.
Etzioni, A. (1986) 'The case for a multiple-utility conception', *Economics and Philosophy* 2:159–83.
Evans, R. W. (1987) letter to *The Lancet*, i:1372.
Hirsch, F. (1977) *Social Limits to Growth*, London: Routledge & Kegan Paul.
Lancaster, K. J. (1971) *Consumer Demand: A New Approach*, New York: Columbia University Press.

Sen, A. K. (1979) 'Personal utilities and public judgements: or what's wrong with welfare economics?', *Economic Journal* 89:537–58. Reprinted in Sen (1982).

Sen, A. K. (1980) 'Equality of what?', in S. McMurrin (ed.) *The Tanner Lectures on Human Values*, Cambridge: Cambridge University Press. Reprinted in Sen (1982).

Sen, A. K. (1982) *Choice, Welfare, and Measurement*, Oxford: Blackwell.

Sen, A. K. (1983) 'Poor, relatively speaking', *Oxford Economic Papers* 35:153–69.

Sen, A. K. (1985) 'A sociological approach to the measurement of poverty – a reply to Professor Peter Townsend', *Oxford Economic Papers* 37:669–76.

Smith, A. (1987) 'Qualms about QALYs', *The Lancet*, i:1134.

Torrance, G. W. (1986) 'Measurement of health state utilities for economic appraisal: a review', *Journal of Health Economics* 5:1–30.

Townsend, P. (1979) *Poverty in the United Kingdom: A Survey of Household Resources and Standards of Living*, Harmondsworth: Penguin.

Townsend, P. (1985) 'A sociological approach to the measurement of poverty – a rejoinder to Professor Amartya Sen', *Oxford Economic Papers* 37:659–68.

Williams, A. (1977) 'Measuring the quality of life of the elderly', in L. Wingo and A. Evans (eds) *Public Economics and the Quality of Life*, Baltimore: Johns Hopkins Press.

Williams, A. (1985) 'Economics of coronary artery bypass grafting', *British Medical Journal* 291:326–9.

Williams, A. (1987) letter to *The Lancet*, i:1372.

Chapter Two

THE QUALITY OF LIFE
Starting from Aristotle

CHRISTOPHER MEGONE

The quality of life is a notion that has been discussed, in various guises, throughout the history of philosophy. In recent times such a notion has been variously employed by social scientists, for example by economists concerned with the question how society should best allocate resources. But how should a measure of quality of life be determined? This paper will draw on some ideas found in Aristotle so as to apply them to the modern discussion.

The paper begins by defending the attempt to shed light on practical issues through the introduction of a theoretical apparatus. Thereafter two main claims are made. One is that any conception of the quality of life taken to be purely empirically grounded will face problems. The second is that any adequate measure of the quality of life should take account of an Aristotelian approach. The first idea is implicit in criticism of a particular measure, the QALY (Quality Adjusted Life Year). This attempts to assess quality of life from the point of view of health status, where health status is then taken as a consideration in determining the allocation of resources for health care. It is a measure characteristic of welfare economics in its fundamentally utilitarian nature. The criticism of this measure serves to motivate the introduction of the Aristotelian line of thought. Aristotle is concerned with the quality of life at a fairly general level, so his remarks can be brought to bear on any such measure, but, as an example, their applicability to the topic of health is briefly indicated.

The term 'quality of life' is ambiguous. On the one hand there is the quality of an individual's life, a reflection of how well his life is going; but there is also a broader concept, capturing roughly the quality of the living conditions around an agent, where these can be picked out independent of how well the agent's own life goes. These living conditions might encompass the environment and culture in (for example) a given society. It may well be that the two notions intersect, that the quality of an individual's life is affected by the quality of his environment and culture, and that these are in part a function of how well the lives of agents in the society go. But the two ideas, which might be termed private and public quality of life, respectively, are certainly distinct. With this distinction made the first issue may be addressed.

'The quality of life' is a grandiose term. The ordinary man (by whom I mean myself) does not often talk in terms of the quality of his life, nor is the quality of life, more generally, a common topic of conversation. So is any investigation of such a concept entirely a theoretical invention, and thus of no use to the problems of the practical world, which need to be solved instead by making use of the concepts in play in that world? There are really two questions here. First, is there any ordinary grip on the concept of quality of life at all, or is it something that those actually facing the problems of health resource allocation, for example, simply do not employ? If the latter were the case, there might be some mismatch between a theoretical solution to a theoretical problem, and the real problem faced by health administrators or doctors, say, – a mismatch due to the former using a concept that the latter have *no* grip on at all. But second, even if there is some fairly standard idea of what quality of life concerns, might it be that any attempt to produce a more refined notion for the purpose of measurement, employing theoretical devices, inevitably distorts from the original? And again the worry is similar. The notion of quality of life is employed by theorists to address certain problems on the basis that those actually facing the problems see this notion as a relevant factor. But if the theorist (any economist, say) solves the problem in terms of a distorted theoretical account of the factor, distorted because the theoretical refinements slant the notion in a certain way – if this is the case, then, it has been suggested, the theorist has not solved the original problem (Mulkay, Ashmore, and Pinch 1987).

The two questions can be dealt with for each interpretation of quality of life in turn. Consider first the quality of an individual's life. Does the ordinary person have a grasp on this notion? Although it is plausible that he does not talk, nor even reflect, employing such a term, it is also plausible that he does have a grasp on it. To grasp the notion of quality of life, it is simply necessary to grasp the application of qualitative terms to one's life; and such talk of life, or of projects which constitute life, as going better or worse, is common enough. Furthermore the reflection that life is going better or worse in the light of health factors is equally common. An individual might well try to decide whether or not to have an operation in terms of its effects on his quality of life. Thus the notion of (private) quality of life is not in itself theoretical. And such a notion is in principle relevant to the application of resources for health, for example.

However it is no doubt true that this ordinary notion of private quality of life is fairly rough. To grasp the term is to grasp the idea of life going better or worse, not to grasp a well fleshed-out account of the good life, or the bad life. But if the term is to appear in a theoretical solution to a problem, if, for example, quality of life is to play a part in assessing the product of a course of action in health care, then a more precise notion may be required. The mere idea of life going better or worse may not be adequate. But if the term is rough, how is a more precise definition to be reached? One solution is that it is to be reached by means of theoretical considerations. But if the theory concerns the nature of the quality of life, where are theoretical considerations to be found except by appeal to the definition? A more general solution is that theory and definition go together; the process of reaching a definition and the process of arriving at a theory are pursued together (see Griffin 1982:332). Thus in this case the fact that quality of life is a matter of degree (a constraint given by the term) together with the need for precise measurement (a constraint given by the aim of the theory) suggest the term must be defined so that numerical assignments may be made to components of quality of life. But then the attribution of such assignments (now part of the definition) may have repercussions for the theory about quality of life – such as the comparability of components of quality of life (e.g. in this case, physical pain and physical disability).

But then, as the second question mentioned asked, is the resultant notion of quality of life, refined by theoretical considerations, quite different from the ordinary notion which is part of the practical problem? This is not obviously so, since it is the original practical problem which has guided the theory and the refinement of the term. The theory aims to produce the best[1] solution to the problem and thus refines the term with that end in mind. But the crucial thing is that this is a *refinement* of the original term. The two must share a core of meaning, and so to that extent mean the same. If the theory is unsatisfactory, the refinement may be likewise. But even here the term will not mean something quite *different*. Given these considerations, the economist, for example, who employs the concept of quality adjusted life years will be using the notion of quality of life in an important sense in the same way as the ordinary person.[2]

The same questions can now be dealt with for the concept of public quality of life. Again it is plausible that such a notion does exist, at least implicitly. (Possibly the explicit use of this notion is more common than the other.) Public choices, such as where to locate an airport, implicitly involve reflection as to better or worse living conditions, hence reflection as to quality of life. And by parity with the reasoning above an attempt to produce a theoretically adequate notion of (public) quality of life must be guided by the ordinary notion (given the problem to which it is relevant), so the theoretical concept will be a refinement of the same concept.

Given these answers, the use of the concept of quality of life as one relevant to the allocation of resources in health care, and the attempt to incorporate it within a theory designed to deal with that question, remains a coherent project, open to reason.

Consider, then, a current attempt in social science to measure quality of life (Williams 1981; Rosser, Kind, and Williams 1982; Williams 1985). The general problem is how best to allocate resources to competing types of health care, given that the resources are finite. A plausible solution involves evaluating each type of health care, and assessing the resources it uses, so as to arrive at a corresponding ratio for each sort. Here quality of life enters in.

One method of assessing the value of health care (say a type of operation) is simply to note the increase in life expectancy it produces. But this seems too restrictive; surely its effect on the quality of life is relevant. It is not merely how long one lives, but the state of one's health over that period that is relevant. On this view, procedures in health care should be ranked in terms of the increase in expected Quality Adjusted Life Years (QALYs) they produce. More accurately, procedures should be ranked so that those that produce more quality adjusted life years (gains in health) per unit of resource take priority over those that produce less (Williams

31

1985:326). Such a view may seem plausible, but it follows that within it there must be some method of assessing the quality of life and this will be the focus of discussion.

The method adopted by Williams *et al.*, is described by him as 'feeling functional', but is essentially the view that quality of life is a function of preference-satisfaction, very similar to the utilitarian idea that welfare is to be cashed out as desire-satisfaction (Williams 1981:273; Griffin 1982:333). Although there are a variety of ideas about how to determine preferences, the view that quality of life is a function of preference-satisfaction seems to be a major strand within the health economics literature.[3] Thus while the Williams method will be used for illustrative purposes, the main target of discussion will be this preference-satisfaction approach. Now consider further the illustration. Williams' method for assessing the quality of life (with respect to health) requires the characterization of a range of states of health in terms of two considerations, degrees of physical disability and degrees of stress. Subjects are then asked to assess the relative values of these states, so described, on a scale in which a normal healthy life has the value '1' while death has the value '0'. The preferences of the community are then arrived at by some process of aggregation which involves the standard problems of inter-personal comparison of scales.[4]

There is a range of problems here, but they fall into two categories, one of which has very general implications, so is addressed first. A central problem for the view related concerns the dimensions (physical disability and stress) in terms of which the states of health are characterized.[5] For the use of such dimensions itself involves evaluation, and evaluation which affects the results. The stipulation of these dimensions entails that the agent's choices between states are made with certain parameters. Thus states of health are characterized in terms of a certain degree of physical disability and a degree of stress, rather than, for example, in terms of the capacity for creativity and employment. Thus agents' preferences will depend on their attitudes to the parameters stipulated, and might well be different if they were to assess the options relative to other parameters. But given that preferences are thus dependent on parameters it becomes very important that the right parameters are picked out. Williams is aware of this problem too, but his response is obscure. He claims that 'the dimensions of health . . . must emerge from empirical investigation in which respondents are permitted to reveal their own constructs of health' (Williams 1981:275). Such constructs are not, presumably, to be treated as preferences, so how are they aggregated? And in any case why is it likely that such constructs will give rise to plausible dimensions of health? (The justification for *this* method is left quite unclear.)

In a similar way, the states which constitute the end points on the scale, the state of being healthy, and to a lesser extent the state of death, are not empirical matters either, but evaluative. (These end-point states are at least formally the same in many of the methods of determining preferences towards health.) Williams claims that the notion of being healthy 'is not one of perfect fitness but that state where society considers someone as to all intents and purposes healthy' (Williams 1981:274), but this is none the less an evaluative notion of good health. The characterization of this state will, pre-sumably, be not unconnected to the way in which other states of health are picked out (see above) but preferential attitudes between this state and other states of health will clearly depend on its descrip-tion. How is this to be selected? Williams states that health as '"normal" functioning' is 'a socially constructed notion' (Williams 1981:274). This is obscure, but once more the idea seems to be that the concept of being healthy should be constructed out of the views of members of society. Again it is not clear quite how such construction takes place. Nor, again, is it at all obvious why this is an appropriate way of establishing what good health is.

In general there might appear to be an unpleasant dilemma for the empirical determination of preferences. Either the options are presented to the chooser without parameters being specified, or parameters are cited. But in the former case it is not clear that dif-ferent agents will have chosen between relevantly similar options, so that there will be an additional worry about aggregating their prefer-ences, while in the latter case the selection of parameters involves evaluation. And that evaluation requires defence.

There may be a further dilemma here. In order to establish the preferences of subjects the investigator needs a proper notion of good health (i.e. some substantive account of what it is) as one of the parameters. But if that exists then the notion of quality of life (with regard to health), the supposed object of investigation, is already given.

The discussion here illustrates a general problem for any social scientist developing a concept of the quality of life – namely that any method which seeks to establish the nature of quality of life by purely empirical means will in fact employ evaluative assumptions.[6] And the method itself will not provide justification for those evaluative assumptions. So in this example the preference-satisfaction approach to quality of life cannot be, even at its core, purely empirical. Given this, there will be less (comparative) implausibility in an (Aristotelian) approach which is, to a degree, non-empirical and evaluative, but seeks to argue for its evaluations. For in being non-empirical and evaluative it stands on precisely the same basis as any rival. And in providing grounds for its evaluations it makes a case for their incorporation within any account put forward in social science.

Before turning to this alternative, there is the second category of problems for the view outlined to consider. These focus on the use made of preferences. First, it has been observed that certain basic assumptions which the investigation makes about interviewees' preferences are implausible (Mulkay, Ashmore, and Pinch 1987). One such assumption is stability, the assumption that individuals' preferences are stable over time. This assumption is necessary if the scale of preferences is to be of use over time. But it has been objected that the assumption is not correct, and indeed Brandt rejects the entire preference-satisfaction approach on the grounds that preferences do change over time but there is 'no ... intelligible programme for weighing desires that change with time' (Brandt 1979: ch. 7; quoted in Griffin 1982:337).

Second, there are conceptual difficulties. To begin with, there is the question whether an agent's desires do reveal his preferences. On the one hand there are well-known points based on attitudes to risk and falsity of beliefs. The agent's choice may vary in line with his attitude to risk as well as his preference. Hence in order to determine his preference from his choice it is necessary to hold some (justified) view of his attitude to risk. Alternatively, the agent's choice may rest on a false belief as well as a preference, so that he chooses the wrong means to his goal. Interpretation of choice therefore involves complexity.

But there is a second deeper point here. Whilst it is obvious that in some sense a person's choices depend on his preferences (there is some kind of semantic relation here) it is not obvious that his preferences comprise or flow from just one kind of thing, namely his assessment of his own good, or expected good (Sen 1977; Culyer 1981). Thus Sen distinguishes two further features, sympathy and commitment of a broadly moral type) which may be reflected in a person's choices (Sen 1977:326–9). His suggestion is that sympathy can be captured within a person's desire – an individual can have sympathetic desires for *another's* good. But commitment cannot (or at least not within first-order desires)[7] – it is of a different nature. Given these distinctions, whilst an individual can only make one choice it is necessary (Sen suggests) to distinguish his interests (based on his desire for his own good), his welfare (including self-interested and sympathetic desires) and his idea of what should be done (including his commitments) (Sen 1977:338). The question then arises as to which of these three is relevant to his quality of life. That in turn raises the question of the connection between private and public quality of life. Is his private quality of life affected by the public quality of life? For the satisfaction of his sympathetic preferences and of his commitments will affect the public realm. This question, whether there are things of value which are not reducible to an individual's values, is passed over here (on this see Waldron 1985).

There is a third problem with preferences, namely that individuals can be mistaken in their desires. They can desire objects not in their interests. Thus satisfying such desires will not improve their quality of life. On one account desires can fail to be rational because based on insufficient information or a failure of logic (Brandt 1979). But even if fully informed an agent can desire objects which are simply not in his interest, he can make some form of cognitive mistake. It is common enough for an individual to pursue a course which he later recognizes not to have been in his interests. And it is widely agreed that certain agents, such as drug addicts, may not be in a position to know their own interest.[8] Given this it is not at all clear why, once an individual's self-interested preferences have been accurately discovered, they should be taken as information relevant to determining the (private) quality of life. In other words, even at the last, when an agent's choices are correctly interpreted, they only reveal that agent's perception of his interests, his values – but why suppose that in this area alone individuals are infallibly right? These specific difficulties may also make an alternative approach attractive.

The alternative approach is Aristotelian, as advertised. The issues it raises are complex and the argument suggested here merely picks out details. It is to be found in the first book of the Nichomachean

35

Ethics (N.E.) (Aristotle 1915) where Aristotle introduces the question of the good life for man and thus is concerned with the (private) quality of life. Once outlined, application of the argument to the measurement of health status in terms of quality of life is indicated, an example of its potential general application.

In N.E. 1,5 Aristotle discusses the popular views that the good life is one of pleasure, or of honour, or of wealth. Each view is dismissed. Pleasure (by which he means some sort of sensory state) captures only the baser instincts of humans. The life of honour depends too much on those bestowing honour; their judgement may be whimsical or temporary (not indices of the good life). Wealth is merely a means, not an end in itself. The remainder of the Ethics is an elaboration of Aristotle's own account of the good life, but it is the immediate next stage that is relevant here. In the seventh chapter of book one, having established that the good life for man is something final and self-sufficient (lacking nothing), he suggests a clearer account might be given 'if we could first ascertain the function of man' (Aristotle 1915). This gives rise to the famous function argument, of which there is another version in the Eudemian Ethics (Woods 1982). There are many questions as to what exactly the structure of the argument is, what it achieves and whether it is valid, but here only the bare bones are required (see further, Woods 1982; Hutchinson 1986). The basic idea is that if a thing has a function, or purpose, then that thing will be achieving its goal, in the best state (so a good example of its kind), when it completely achieves that function or purpose. For example, if a washing machine's purpose is to wash clothes, then a good washing machine washes clothes well. Thus if a human being has a function, or purpose (simply *as* a human being), then he will be in the best state when that purpose is achieved. If man's purpose is a kind of life, as it plausibly is, then his living the good life will consist in his achieving that purpose. In sum, if we can discover what man's purpose is, we can discover what the good life for man is.

What then is man's function? In the course of the account in N.E. 1,7 Aristotle suggests that it is *rational activity*. From this it follows that the good life for man is the fully (or perfect) rational active life. But how does Aristotle establish that this is the function of human beings? Once more this is a complicated issue of which only bare bones are needed (see further, Megone 1988). Aristotle's views flow from his general theory of natural kinds, of which human beings are

36

an example. He holds that in the case of natural kinds there is a connection between the essence of a member of the kind (what it is to be that thing) and the thing's function. The connection between the essence and function is that the essence explains the thing's characteristic behaviour, and explains it as the thing's *purpose*, what the thing is (metaphorically) meant to do, so what a good example of the kind will do. Roughly speaking, Aristotle's idea is that in the natural world a large number of occurrences are regular (this does not mean statistically most common) and cyclical, and these regular occurrences which are exclusive to a thing, or part of its regular cycle of behaviour and serving to sustain the recurrence of that cycle, are to be explained by reference to the object's essence. And the explanation is purposive or, technically, teleological. Thus a thing's function is that state, or set of activities, which can be explained teleologically by reference to the essence.

The idea, then, is that the explanation of aspects of a thing's behaviour may be given by reference to the kind of thing it is. Two brief examples may help. The explanation why an animal is stalking its prey in a certain way is given by citing its being a lion. The explanation why a plant has trapped a fly is that it is a Venus fly-catcher. These explanations are teleological. By contrast the plant's leaves being brown with mould cannot be so explained.

This rapid account can now be summarized. Aristotle holds that the best state of an object is the fulfilment of its function, or purpose, which, in the case of a member of a natural kind, is its characteristic or regular behaviour. But for natural-kind members the function is explained (teleologically) by its essence. Hence that state which is the best state of an object is explained (teleologically) by its essence. The reason *why* such a state is the best state is that the creature belongs to such and such a kind. Thus a clearer account of the good life for man will rest ultimately (via man's function) on man's essence. Aristotle suggests that man's definition is rational animal (Aristotle 1928) so that the essence of man is the capacity for rational action. The definition is plausible in the light of man's characteristic activities which are distinctively rational. It is plausible that a thing defined by its capacity for rational action should have such activities as its purpose. And given this definition, the good life for man will be a fully rational active life.

It is important to note here that such a definition is not intel-lectualist, hence does not entail a peculiarly intellectual account of the good life. Man is defined by the capacity for reasoning. This is the sense of rational according to which man is rational and amoebae are not. Amoebae do not act for reasons, whilst human beings do. Thus (intentional) human action is distinguished as being for reasons. Thus the good life for man need not be one of pure contemplation, but can include virtuous behaviour which is, say, practically rational.

The important upshot from all this is that the good life for man, hence, in modern terms, an account of the factors relevant to the (private) quality of life, derives from an account of human nature.

How then does the approach aid our example, health status measurement? What follows is the beginning of an answer.

Suppose that Aristotle is correct in his account of the essence of man as a rational animal. This account has two components, it picks man out as an animal, with the differentiating feature of the capacity for reason. As an animal man will move or behave; as a rational animal he will be capable of pure reason or behaviour governed by reasons – actions. Thus the good life for man will involve perfectly rational activity of these two sorts. Since the exercise of reason is in an important sense up to the individual, how well a life goes will likewise be in an important sense up to the individual. Thus health will not be directly a component of the good life, unless being healthy is intrinsically good for an animal, but rather a necessary condition for the attainment of the good life. The account of essence will determine dimensions of health indirectly, by picking out those dimensions necessary to allow the living of a good life.

So what dimensions of health status measurement might the account suggest? It seems clear that the capacity to reason is important to the quality of life. Thus operations, or health care, which sustain or improve this capacity will be important to quality of life. This obviously includes work on or related to the brain's functioning, but more generally the areas of mental health. If the parameters in our earlier example of QALY analysis are recalled, namely physical disability and stress, this criterion seems not to be included at all. (This depends in part on what exactly stress comes to.) Furthermore, the relevance of physical disability to quality of life will depend on the importance of physical ability first for the performance of practically rational activities such as virtuous action, and second for the performance of satisfying human animal activities such as sport, conversation and so on. Thus in the first case it is plausible that physical manoeuvrability is necessary for certain types of courage, not others, perhaps not necessary for acts of unselfishness, thoughtfulness, integrity. In the second case, manoeuvrability is clearly important for sport, but not for conversation. What these rudimentary thoughts suggest is both the possibility of rather different dimensions of health status and, second, a theoretical framework within which to forge more precise characterizations of those dimensions. Thus, with regard to the latter, it might be hoped that as well as indicating the extent to which physical disability is a factor relevant to health status at all, the theory might provide grounds for suggestions as to the importance of types of physical disability given the types of activity which they hinder.

Despite the suggestions here, which constitute only a beginning, it might be that the Aristotelian approach would not produce markedly different results from certain types of preference-satisfaction theory. However, at least two important differences would remain. First, by grounding an account of quality of life in an account of human nature the theory suggests that the components of health status are fixed, not subject to change as human preferences change. Of course the components would change given a different view of human nature, but the components are in principle fixed by whatever is the correct account of what it is to be a human being. By contrast, given that preferences are changeable, an account attaching components of health status to them implies the components are intrinsically changeable. The second difference is that the Aristotelian approach provides a grounding for the evaluations of health arrived at, as opposed to incorporating ungrounded evaluations, hence is not open to some of the charges raised against its rival earlier. In other areas of social science the substantive effects might be more significant. But, at a minimum, the two points mentioned above will be of general application.

NOTES

1 *Best outright*, not relative to some set of considerations.
2 Apparently contra Mulkay, Ashmore, and Pinch (1987:13). Relatedly, the economist's (or anyone's) efforts to show he has the right theory will be a case of providing reasons, not mere persuasion (contra Mulkay, Ashmore and Pinch 1987:33–5).

3 Various methods for determining preferences are described in Culyer 1980. Elsewhere (Culyer 1981:6) it appears that even experts' valuations are incorporated as preferences, where incorporated at all.
4 Williams is aware of these problems (Williams 1981:276), but does not provide any satisfactory solution.
5 Mulkay, Ashmore, and Pinch (1987:26) make a slightly different point on correspondence. They query how plausible it is that individuals do evaluate their ordinary conception of quality of life in terms of the discussions offered. But the point here is that even if agents can quite easily do this, their preferences might be different if other dimensions were used. Hence the choice of dimensions is importantly evaluative.
6 These go well beyond those mentioned in Williams (1981), or in general in the literature I have seen. The problem will be more apparent as attempts are made to refine QALY measuring devices by introducing further parameters.
7 'It might be captured by orderings of desire – first order, second order . . .' (Sen 1977:336–9).
8 Though I think such remarks are best accounted for by realism about values, this issue does not turn on that question. Even an anti-realist like Blackburn tries to account for mistakes about values (Blackburn 1970).

REFERENCES

Aristotle (1915) 'Nichomachean Ethics', in W. D. Ross (ed.) *The Works of Aristotle*, vol. 9, London: O.U.P.
Aristotle (1928) 'Topics', in W. D. Ross (ed.) *The Works of Aristotle*, vol. 1, London: O.U.P.
Blackburn, S. (1970) 'Moral Realism', in J. Casey (ed.)
Brandt, R. (1979) *A Theory of the Right and the Good*, Oxford: Clarendon Press.
Culyer, A. J. (1980) 'Needs, values and health status measurement', in A. J. Culyer and K. G. Wright (eds) *Economic Prospects of Health Services*, London: Martin Robertson.
Culyer, A. J. (1981) 'Health, economics and health economics', in J. Van der Gaag and M. Perlman (eds) *Health, Economics and Health Economics*, Leiden: North Holland.
Griffin, J. (1982) 'Modern utilitarianism', *Revue Internationale de Philosophie* 141:331–75.
Hutchinson, D. S. (1986) *The Virtues of Aristotle*, London: Routledge.
Megone, C. B. (1988) 'Aristotle on essentialism and natural kinds, Physics II:1' forthcoming.
Mulkay M., Ashmore, M., and Pinch, T. (1987) 'Measuring the quality of life – of sociological invention concerning the application of economics to health care' (manuscript).
Rosser, R., Kind, P., and Williams, A. (1982) 'The value of the quality of life: psychometric evidence', in M. W. Jones-Lee (ed.) *The Value of Life and Safety*, Leiden: North Holland.

Sen, A. K. (1977) 'Rational fools: a critique of the behavioural foundations of economic theory', *Philosophy and Public Affairs* 6:317–44.

Waldron, J. (1985) 'Rights, welfare and public choice', paper delivered to Ethics and Economics Conference, University of York.

Williams, A. (1981) 'Welfare economics and health status measurement', in J. Van der Gaag and M. Perlman (eds) *Health, Economics and Health Economics*, Leiden; North Holland.

Williams, A. (1985) 'Economics of coronary artery bypass grafting', *British Medical Journal* 291:326–9.

Woods, M. (1982) *Aristotle's Eudemian Ethics, Books 1, 2, and 8*, Oxford: Clarendon Press.

Chapter Three

THE QUALITY OF LIFE

A contrast between utilitarian and existentialist approaches[1]

JOANNA HODGE

> The other possible reaction, in ten year's time, might be to say
> that we should stop pussyfooting around in this business and
> launch a massive social survey to get some really representative
> data on a large number of people (100,000?)[2]

The point of setting up a contrast between utilitarian and existential
approaches to discussing and attempting to measure quality of life is
to identify the strengths and limits of quality of life measurement in
allocating health resources. By setting up an alternative frame of
enquiry, the existential, it becomes possible to identify some of the
limiting assumptions at work within the utilitarian tradition in
which such welfare issues are discussed. This then reveals how those
assumptions both make possible the discussion and limit the kind of
results which that enquiry can produce. The point is not to reject
out of hand all enquiries set up within the utilitarian frame, merely
to point out that some of the dilemmas in health care may be the
result of the limits on what can be analysed within that frame. The
argument then is threefold: to show the strengths and limits of the
utilitarian frame; to show that sometimes an alternative frame,
constructed by reference to existentialism, may be useful; and to
show thereby that the hope of making use of a single analytical
frame in order to resolve all the questions posed by health care is a
mistake.

The philosophical preconditions for hypothesizing in terms of
such an analytical frame are worth examining. Adorno and
Horkheimer[3] argue that there is a close connection between the
growth of fascistic social organization and the positing of an all-
encompassing system of values and goals for society. They argue

that the eighteenth-century dream of a single rationality through which the conflicts and difficulties of human living might be resolved has turned into a system of administration in which people become bearers of social roles, not individuals with self-determination, and in which people are continually confronted with the necessity of accommodating to external requirements, rather than given the space to develop a sense of autonomy. This administrative interference then undermines the development of autonomy and self-determination in individuals. The suggestion that there is a need for complementary and mutually incompatible frames of reference is then a challenge to the dream of such all-encompassing values and goals, and is potentially, at least, a site of resistance to increasing authoritarianism. If there is no single, obviously superior programme for the resolution of human conflicts, then there must be discussion, negotiation, and tentativeness in the manner in which any programme is put forward. Such tentativeness is of itself a form of resistance to an increase in authoritarianism, and the suggestion made here, that it is necessary to shift between mutually incompatible frames of reference, is intended in the spirit of that anti-fascist tentativeness.[4]

It is characteristic of a particular kind of philosophical practice, not of all philosophy, to suppose that decision making can be given a rational foundation in theoretical enquiry. It is characteristic of a particular kind of theory of society to suppose that it forms a single process, of which a unified account can be given. Those two great Victorians, Mill and Marx, are committed to both positions, and they therefore share a philosophical frame of reference. Both thought it possible to produce global solutions to the problems of human societies, which could be deduced from principles and justified in terms of the values endorsed by their enquiries: for Mill, liberty and choice; for Marx, fairness and need. For Mill the central measure of value is utility, for Marx it is work; but for both there is a single measure. Their arguments in the end rest on contrasting presumptions about what human beings need to flourish, and on contrasting accounts of what human beings are like.

Such accounts of human beings are, however, clearly contestable, and for existential philosophy any such general prescriptions about what it is to be human subvert the self-determination, which is for existentialism the defining characteristic of what it is to be human. Nietzsche and Sartre, Kierkegaard and Heidegger all dispute the possibility of providing a single measure of value and a single account of what human beings need to flourish. In their work, there are to be found three further reasons why this model of deducing policies for social improvement from first principles is dubious: first, that a total account of the problems cannot be given; second, that a set of principles producing a single resolution is not available; and third, that the very model of constructing a set of theoretical criteria for decisions and then proceeding to decision making is a model which postpones indefinitely the making of decisions. Existentialism puts into question all four of these elements, and is thus in opposition to both Mill's liberalism and to Marx's socialism.

In practical matters, both Mill and Marx tend to accept the necessity of selecting the best of the available options, rather than deducing decisions about action from first principles. They and the political practices emerging from their work hover uncertainly between a Platonic idealism, with a rigorous deduction of consequences from first principles, and an Aristotelian pragmatism, as indeed do the works of both Aristotle and Plato. There is an implicit authoritarianism in such rigorous deduction, and both the Marxian party and the role of the enlightened intellectual in liberalism are suspect to those committed to pluralism and consultation. The party members and the intellectuals tend to see themselves as best qualified to set up the first principles, draw the conclusions, and impose them on societies, irrespective of the wishes of the actual populations. Existentialism implies a surrender of an illusory hope of providing ultimate justifications for a particular social order and for social policy. The diversity and hesitations surrounding the political allegiances of Sartre and Nietzsche are confirmation of this surrender. Contrasting existentialism to liberalism and Marxism then reveals a curious complicity between the latter two with respect to this model of producing and justifying social policy, and with respect to the authoritarianism implied in supposing that there are complete coherent resolutions of the tensions of human societies.

There are four key assumptions at work in QALY measurement, in cost-benefit analysis, in utilitarianism, and in the British empirical tradition which provides the conceptual framework for these three. These assumptions are: that my identity remains constant irrespective of psychological and physiological trauma; that my identity is somehow given in advance of such states; that my death is an external limit on my flourishing, not an integral part of my daily living; and that there is an objective scale of preferences, which can be rationally constructed, concerning the desirability and undesirability of physical states.[5] All these assumptions rest on one basic assumption, which is central to utilitarianism, to liberalism, to humanism: that there is a basic structure, called human nature, which constitutes our similarity to each other, permits comparisons between us, and provides the basis for our identities. In any rigorous discussion of humanism, of liberalism, indeed of utilitarianism, this assumption, basic though it is to their coherence, is always put in question. It is certainly put in question by John Stuart Mill, in his essays 'On Liberty' and 'Utilitarianism', which provide a point of departure for contemporary British thinking on liberalism and the value of life.

Mill also recognizes that not everyone has the same preferences, and that some will judge the preferences of others to be not only inferior to their own, but actually damaging to the possessor of those preferences. It is for this reason that education has such an enormously important role in liberalism, and certainly in the liberalism of Mill, since it is recognized that people acquire their preferences, they are not born with them; that preferences are alterable, they are not fixed once for all; and that a given order of preferences may not in fact be in the best interests of health and well-being of the person holding them. Thus addiction is a problem precisely because someone has a preference for something which is not only damaging and wasteful of their health and energy, but also subsequently becomes damaging to others and wasteful of their resources, both financial and emotional. This lays the basis for a difference between liberal natural rights theory and utilitarianism, since for the latter, it is possible to construe the preferences of an individual as detrimental to that individual, such that society is licensed to intervene. Marxism expands this to supposing that not only may individual preferences be harmful, but the values endorsed by individuals and by collectives may be harmful as well.

The epigraph to this paper quotes Williams' proposal for amassing empirical evidence on individual preferences concerning the allocation of resources. The problem is that while a survey will give us a sense of community values, sometimes it may be important to override these values. Just because the mass of the population is in favour of hanging or opposed to homosexuals openly holding high office is no reason to suppose that these are morally founded or

economically efficient requirements. Everyone has their own prejudice and blindness; mine is impatience with spending on fertility
programmes. Just because a prejudice is held by a majority is no
grounds for turning that prejudice into a principle guiding decision
making. The resources which would go into producing such a
survey should perhaps rather go into health education, which would
in any case be a necessary precondition if respondents are to be in a
position to make informed choices about the available treatments
and their consequences, as indeed Williams points out.[6] A further
difficulty with such surveys is that the views of those consulted are in
all likelihood not internally consistent, nor indeed stable. The
chances are that as a result of taking part in such a survey the views
of many of the participants may change, become more or perhaps
less confused. In any case, the results will not reflect the given views
of those consulted, but the views to which they are moving. The
problem here is the assumption that people and their views are fixed
and unalterable, rather than in process of constitution, and particularly liable to change if confronted with difficult, complicated
decisions.

While this survey would establish the preferences of real people,
in calculating QALYs it is not actual human beings or actual conditions which are in question, it is hypothetical cases and their
corresponding costs and benefits, taken without reference to the
context in which any actual individual finds themselves. Thus there
is a gap between the abstract individuals, in terms of whom QALY
calculation takes place, and the actual individuals who are offered or
denied treatments on the basis of that calculation. QALY calculation considers benefit to a particular kind of individual of a particular treatment, in terms of individual mobility and experience of
pain. Another possible frame of reference for decisions about allocating resources, as with discussions of the value of life,[7] would be
the costs to the community of not pursuing the treatment, and that
of course involves considering the social costs of non-functioning:
old people ceasing to be able to look after themselves, and people
with primary care responsibilities ceasing to be able to perform
them. This model would then concentrate on the costs of non-
treatment and take them into account in decisions about the allocation of resources in health care. The problem then is that existing
inequalities in wage-earning power and supposed value to the
community have to be critically assessed, such that cabinet

ministers and wage earners with dependants do not automatically get preferential treatment, on the basis of their supposed indispensability. This poses the problem of the effects on decision making of existing social values. The contrast here is between assessing costs and benefits in terms of hypothetical individuals, and assessing them in a community context.

The point of contrasting utilitarianism and existentialism is not to show one right and the other wrong, but to show that choices of value are being made in the choice of frame of reference, that assumptions are being made which are not indisputable. These assumptions may turn out to be advantageous indeed indispensable for the purposes of particular kinds of enquiry, but they cannot be rationally grounded beyond all question. The contrast makes it possible to discuss the relation between social and individual values. There are three significant differences between the two traditions, the utilitarian and the existential. There is, first, a difference about the nature of goodness and a correlative difference about what constitutes health; second, a difference concerning the relation between personal identity, life, and death; and third, a difference concerning the relation between the individual, identity, and value. The two traditions undoubtedly make incompatible claims, since utilitarianism presupposes and existentialism puts in doubt the possibility of methodological individualism.

For Mill, the good should not be conceived as some unattainable ideal set up against actual human experience, with the effect of making human activity seem doomed to failure; nor should it be understood as an abstraction to which all human beings, by virtue of their rational capacities, have access. The good is a realizable goal, to be defined by collective negotiation. In this he and Marx are in agreement. The two models of how to get to that human good are those of individual choice in a free market, and of central planning in terms of human need. In the case of health provision, and probably more generally, neither model can in fact function in practice without drawing on the resources of the other. It is necessary to be concerned with both choice and need; it is necessary to combine elements of free market mechanisms and elements of central planning. Theoretical purity is probably not viable in any context, and particularly not in the case of health care. Thus setting up the two models as essentially opposed is a mistake. Indeed both are concerned with aggregation and measurement, with the calculation of values rendered commensurable by means of an arbitrary scale, in Marx's case, work, in Mill's case, utility. This joint emphasis on measurement, and the silence with respect to justifying the standard, marks a difference between liberalism and Marxism on the one hand, and, on the other, existentialism, which does not seek to quantify, and therefore has no need of an arbitrary scale. It therefore has no axioms for which it has no arguments. Correlatively it surrenders the possibility of deducing binding consequences from first principles.

For utilitarianism, and for the practices of cost benefit analysis and welfare calculation which arise out of it, the good is defined as a summation of individual goods, minus the summation of individual harms. Thus there are supposed to be a set of clear distinctions between pleasure and pain, for classical utilitarianism; between cost and benefit, for public finance considerations; between sickness and health, for health care. All these distinctions are brought into question in existentialism. The utilitarian account of the good does have the advantage of being an immanentist definition of good which, for all its faults, has the virtue of making the good open to inspection. Mill and Nietzsche are united against construing the good as some transcendent abstraction. Mill supposes such a conception to be diversionary in setting up a consolation for everyday ills, which a conception of collective welfare can be used to eradicate. Nietzsche argues that conceptions of the good as transcendent in and of itself produces an unhappiness and paralysis of the will, producing unhealthy individuals and sick societies.

In existentialism there is also a suspicion of transcendent accounts of the good, but this is a part of suspicion of any generalized account of the good. Notions of the good in existentialism are construed as products of a complicated network of forces, held in play between different temporal emanations of the self, in its interactions with others, with the world, and with its ideals. The existential account of the good is inseparable from the existential account of identity, and therefore must be held over for discussion. The utilitarian account then is superior in terms of its definiteness and inspectability; the existential account perhaps has the vices of its virtues — its richness and suggestiveness is obtained at the cost of a correlative vagueness. The main problem with the utilitarian conception of the good is that it tends to reduce well-being to a summation of physical conditions, since they are more easily identifiable and comparable. This leads to the science fiction vision of Aldous Huxley's *Brave New World*, in which the primary goal of social activity is reducing frustration and discontent by administering drugs.

Correlative with these divergences around the concept of goodness, there are divergences around the concept of health. Just as the utilitarian account of the good is starkly operational, demonstrating the desirability of specific social and legal reforms and making possible its use in social decision-making processes, so the conception of health which functions within the utilitarian tradition is one which focuses on measurable components in the network of ideas suggested by the notion of health. It is much easier to measure the capacity to walk a mile, than the desire to do so; it is easier to measure physical components in health than it is to measure psychological distress, and environmental and social effects. The desire to measure, indeed the necessity of measuring and comparing outcomes itself prioritizes those aspects of the situation which are less objectively determinate and correlatively less amenable to measurement.

Nietzsche destabilizes the boundaries between sickness and health, between psychological and physical health, between individual and social well-being and pathology. Both physical and psychological sickness are for Nietzsche preconditions for embarking on a task of cultural criticism, for criticizing oversimplifications in understanding and identifying when prejudice and tradition are masquerading as absolute value. Nietzsche already has an account of a mechanism whereby social relations and distributions of power can make people physically ill, or make them appear ill when in fact they are not. Individual pathology and social pathology are then, for Nietzsche, closely linked. Heidegger develops this thought into a critique of a social structure systematically impoverishing the people who live within it. In the 1950s he developed a critique of contemporary society by identifying dehumanizing effects of what he calls the technological insistence on measurability: the very attempt to quantify and control, in his view, leads to an absolute loss of quality in lived experience. This view is put forward in *The Question Concerning Technology and Other Essays* (1977). His argument then would be that the very attempt to measure quality of life is destructive of what it attempts to measure. Here the concerns of QALY measurement and a philosophical concern with what counts as a properly human existence come adrift from one another.

There is confirmation of this in the distress caused to respondents to surveys about their probable reactions to hypothetical health crises. Anxiety induced by considering future ill health is a phenomenon considered by Brooks (1986).[8] Such a phenomenon can be a surprise only to those who assume that knowledge can never have negative effects. Mill puts a great deal of energy into trying to prove that, however much it may appear as though there are costs attached to attaining knowledge, in the long run it is always beneficial. Nietzsche, by contrast, explicitly recognizes that knowledge has above all the negative effect of paralyzing the will, by making available too much information, and giving too great an awareness of the unpredictability of outcomes. Furthermore, for Nietzsche, health is inseparable from self-determination: if you are not self-determining you cannot be healthy. Thus Heidegger and Nietzsche would resist the attempt to separate out consideration of particular physiological and psychological conditions from an overall account of social processes, refusing the strict separation of level between individual states and social process which QALY calculation presupposes.

It has often been noted that in discussing QALYs there is an assumption that death is the null point, that there are conditions worse than death, but that death itself cannot be desirable. This assumption makes suicide necessarily an irrational choice, and makes the suicides of Socrates and of Japanese Samurai simply incomprehensible. This incomprehension is possible only in a profoundly secularized society, in which honour and life after death are not taken seriously. A whole tradition stretching from Socrates, through Plato and Christianity, to Cardinal Newman is thus written off by the rationalizations of utilitarianism. In this secularized context the Christian Science position, which refuses medical intervention as a blasphemy of divine providence, appears strange, and this is an index of the alienness of putting more emphasis on spiritual well-being than on physical health. Energy now goes into the promotion of health and physical well-being, into hospitals, sport, and health manuals, where in previous centuries the emphasis would rather have been on the spiritual, the building of churches and the production of manuals for spiritual guidance. While there is now the medical expertise to correct physical malfunctioning in a way previously inconceivable, this of itself does not guarantee an improvement in terms of this other standard of quality of life.

There are then two models of identity, both of which are challenged by existentialism. There is the liberal conception of identity constituted in advance of any engagement in social process, such that the norms of that process can be deduced by negotiation between those individuals. The natural rights liberal then conceives of some implicit contract between these hypothetical people, for example on the model proposed by John Rawls.[9] The utilitarian conceives of aggregating those individuals' preferences as the means of deducing the norms for collective practice. In both these models identity is conceived as constituted in advance of social practices. There is an alternative, Christian model of identity, which in effect supposes that identity is only finally constituted in God's judgement at the moment of death. Identity, according to this model, is constituted retrospectively. Curiously the Marxian account of identity is more akin to the Christian one than to the model of preconstitution, since human beings acquire full humanity only in a properly socialist society.

The existential account of identity refuses both the constitution of identity in advance and the constitution of identity in retrospect. Identity in the existentialist frame is constituted and reconstituted through the daily decisions and responses produced by individual human beings. A living process and the finitude of human existence are essential determinations of whatever identity is then put in process. The existentialist account of identity refuses to accept a fixity in identity. Identity is constituted for each individual as a process of interaction between external circumstances, responses to those circumstances, and a process of self-determination within those twofold constraints.

For existentialism mortality is a feature of human existence, it is not just a limit point separating bearable from unbearable states. It is a feature of human existence to which each individual must construct a relation. This theme is portrayed in Tolstoy's *The Death of Ivan Illich*. For each individual the relation to death is distinct, and for the community death is an event for which each individual requires preparation. There is some confirmation of this in the concern of nineteenth-century co-operative societies, providing the means by which to provide for funerals. Funerals plainly do not serve the interests of the dead, but rather serve the interests of those mourning and, more importantly in this context, the interests of those mourners as individuals who themselves have to die. Only where death is conceived as an external limit on existence, rather than as a part of that existence, are choices abut where and how to die of no account. Fear of death is of course only exacerbated by an inability to talk about death; and by the unavailability of a language in which to conceive of death.

Even without the extreme case of some people ending up dead as a result of an allocation of resources, it is still the case that some of the people before and after allocation have radically altered states. According to existentialism, I am not the same person before and after confronting the reality of pain and my own death. In *Being and Time* (1927), Heidegger argues that a concern for identity arises from such a confrontation, and that the individual is not in fact separable from the values he/she puts on certain outcomes. Someone leading a pleasant life will be more risk averse than someone leading a miserable one, in terms either of material or mental well-being. On some scales this would suggest that the resources should be put into extending the life of the person who values it, but conversely it might rather suggest that resources should be put into the life seen as not worthwhile in order to make it seem worthwhile to that person. There is a problem in treating health care as an isolated concern when in fact the lives and deaths of individuals are in question, and circumstances occur in which fundamental changes of values and priorities may take place.

For the existentialist model of identity, constitutive of any identity are the values by which that individual lives, and which inform the individual's decisions about what to do, how to treat others, where to invest energy. Identifying that those values are chosen, not given, and that identity is a process for which the individual must take responsibility are for Heidegger, and possibly for Nietzsche, preconditions for an individual having an identity at all. In the absence of these two conditions, the individual is merely a function of existing values, not an individual with an identity, with autonomy, with freedom. The existentialist model then proposes an account of identity, in which the identities of each individual are dissimilar, while sharing a single general structure, whereas utilitarianism offers an account of all individuals as essentially similar. The problem which the existentialist model throws up is that the same individual may have a sequence of identities as a result of radical shifts in orientation and evaluation of priorities. This disrupts the

model of consulting people in advance of physiological and psychological trauma in order to establish what their preferences for their
own treatment would be, although of course the model can still
operate to establish what people in advance of those states judge the
best outcome. The results of such consultation cannot have binding
force even on those individuals when they are later confronted with
the trauma itself, still less do they have binding force on others.

There is then a difference between choosing between options
within a single frame of values, and choosing between value frames.
Choosing between value frames is constitutive of identity, and it is
this theme which existentialism addresses so powerfully. Utilitarianism and the formation of utility functions presuppose a precon-
stituted identity, and presuppose a choice of value frame. Plainly
there are circumstances in which an individual is confronted with a
choice between options, within a given value frame, but the kinds of
concern which are in play in the discussion of QALYs are not just to
do with clearly defined options, but also to do with setting up the
value frame in terms of which options present themselves. There are
choices to be made about what count as lives worth living, about
what kind of people and what kind of world there should be:
making decisions about value, not choosing between equally available options. Existentialism addresses the latter kind of decision
whereas utilitarianism addresses the former kind of choice in a
context where the existential decisions have already been made.
This makes utilitarianism much more useful for the purposes of
resource allocation, but makes its claim as an enquiry about value
much less well-founded than the claim of existentialism to the same
title.

The major problem with utilitarianism is that it illegitimately
presupposes that individuals can make existential decisions once
and for all, and that those choices are not constrained by existing
social values. It presupposes that those decisions set up a value
frame and social context in which it makes sense to plan in terms of
a single coherent social process. The value frame crucially affects
what kind of social process there is and, by refusing to address how
individual decisions and social values change and affect each other,
it becomes impossible to criticize the frame in terms of which policy
is formed and difficult to assess the values endorsed by individuals
and societies. The major problem with these objections is that if
there is to be any social planning at all, these illegitimate pre-

suppositions must be made some of the time. Social planning will be less authoritarian and more humane, if the illegitimacy of these presuppositions is recognized and the requirement continually to discuss and renegotiate values taken seriously.

NOTES

1 The author would like to thank Christine Godfrey and Carol Propper for their helpful comments and suggestions.
2 From Alan Williams: 'Measuring quality of life', printed as ch. 15, pp. 200–10, in George Teeling Smith (ed.): *Health Economics: Prospects for the Future* (Croom Helm, 1987).
3 See *Dialectic of Enlightenment* (1944). While Adorno and Horkheimer appear to share concerns with the existentialist thinking of Heidegger and Sartre, Adorno criticizes both Heidegger and Sartre, Heidegger for his impenetrable language and covert support for fascism, in *Jargon of Authenticity* (RKP, 1973), and Sartre for the arbitrary individualism of his account of the possibility of resisting fascism, in his essay 'Commitment' in *Aesthetics and Politics* (Verso, 1977).
4 For suggestions on the connection between ways of thinking and fascist social tendencies, see the introduction by M. Foucault to G. Deleuze and F. Guattari: *Anti-Oedipus: Capitalism and Schizophrenia* (Viking, 1977).
5 Derek Parfit in *Reasons and Persons* (1984) puts forward arguments to undermine belief in the first two of these assumptions.
6 See article cited in note 2.
7 See Brooks: *The Development and Construction of Health Status Measures: An Overview of the Literature* (Swedish Institute for Health Economics: Report 1986:4).
8 See E. J. Mishan: 'Consistency in the valuation of life' in Frankel Paul, Miller and Paul (eds) *Ethics and Economics* (Blackwell, Oxford, 1985) and A. McGuire and G. Mooney: 'Back to life: resurrecting the value of life debate', Health Economics Research Unit discussion paper no. 05/85, (University of Aberdeen, 1985).
9 See J. Rawls: *The Theory of Justice* (1971).

Part Two

METHODOLOGY

INTRODUCTION
What are QALYs?

PAUL KIND, CLAIRE GUDEX, and CHRISTINE GODFREY

Consideration of alternative forms of treatment for individual patients or health-care programmes for population subgroups, has, in the past, been dominated by the question of survival. Improved life expectancy, regardless of its quality or the cost of securing it, was interpreted as sufficient basis for treatment. Treatments are not, however, always wholly beneficial or free of undesirable consequences. Over the past decade, there has been growing interest in the application of measures which seek to combine information on life expectancy with complementary information on the quality of that life (Weinstein and Stason 1977, 1985; Kaplan *et al.* 1984; Williams 1985), and hence in the concept of quality adjusted life years, or QALYs. Many of the chapters in the book refer to this concept and its use. The purpose of this contribution is to provide a short description of the QALY as implemented in research at the University of York. This introduction to the section on methodology is intended to provide a background to the chapters by Hirst and by Kind (which examine the wider aspects of the measurement of life quality), and to the contribution of Loomes and McKenzie (which outlines a number of criticisms of existing measures). Issues involved in the practical application of QALYs in health care are discussed by Gudex in Part Four.

The QALY is the arithmetic product of life expectancy and an adjustment for the quality of the remaining life years gained. It is important to distinguish between the measurement of life expectancy and the measurement of quality of life. The first requires simple observation whereas the second requires specific instruments designed for the task. Whilst survival data are often easily accessible, quality of life data are not routinely recorded. Even when quality of life data are available, they need to be classified in some way.

In work undertaken at the University of York the quality of life data have been expressed in terms of a classification first put forward by Rosser in research published in the 1970s (Rosser and Watts 1972). This classification has two components: a set of standard *descriptions* of illness states and an associated set of *valuations* from different groups of subjects.

DESCRIPTIONS

Rosser proposed a set of descriptions of states of illness for use in measuring hospital output (Rosser and Watts 1972). She developed her classification using material generated by small groups of doctors. They were asked to describe the criteria they used to decide on the severity of illness in patients. They were asked quite specifically to consider only the present state of the patient; any prognostic implications were to be excluded. Diagnosis was rejected from the outset as being too complex for the purposes of describing patient's severity of illness. Two principal components of severity ultimately emerged from these discussions – observed disability (loss of function and mobility) and subjective distress. All other aspects of the patient's condition were thought to be subsumed within this framework. This descriptive system was used to classify an initial set of 40 patients and subsequent refinement was made following discussion of the results with groups of doctors. The system which was eventually agreed comprised 8 levels of disability and 4 levels of distress (see Table 1).

A second, separate attempt to generate a classification of illness severity was conducted with non-medical subjects. Groups of economists and health administrators were asked to recall two individuals whom they considered to be ill, and two individuals thought to be healthy. The characteristics which differentiated ill and healthy individuals were then listed. The most frequently cited characteristics related to disability (impaired mobility and function) and distress (pain). Rosser concluded that both medical and non-medical reference groups supported similar classification systems.

The descriptions of health states which had emerged from Rosser's consensus exercise with her colleagues were tested. Doctors' ratings of patients were examined to see whether they could use these descriptions to categorize patients reliably, accurately, and quickly. The disability/distress classification was incorporated into a study of patients admitted to a teaching hospital over a one-month period (Rosser and Watts 1972). A total of 2,120 patients were rated on admission by some 50 collaborating doctors from a wide variety of specialities, including ENT, Gynaecology, Urology, Ophthalmology, Psychiatry, as well as General Medicine and Surgery.

VALUATIONS

Rosser's descriptions, as displayed in Table 1, allow 8 levels of disability and 4 levels of distress. Combinations of these two dimensions describe the states of illness. It was considered that an unconscious patient (disability VIII) would experience no distress, hence combinations with other distress levels (B–D) were excluded, leaving 29 states of illness. So that these illness states could be expressed in numeric as well as in a descriptive form Rosser conducted a series of structured interviews with 70 subjects with different current health experiences. Six widely dispersed states of the 29 disability/

Table 1   Rosser's classification of illness states

DISABILITY		DISTRESS	
I.	No disability.	A.	No distress
II.	Slight social disability.	B.	Mild
III.	Severe social disability and/or slight impairment of performance at work.	C.	Moderate
	Able to do all housework except very heavy tasks.	D.	Severe
IV.	Choice of work or performance at work very severely limited.		
	Housewives and old people able to do light housework only, but able to go out shopping.		
V.	Unable to undertake any paid employment.		
	Unable to continue any education.		
	Old people confined to home except for escorted outings and short walks and unable to do shopping.		
	Housewives able only to perform a few simple tasks.		
VI.	Confined to chair or to wheelchair or able to move around in the house only with support from an assistant.		
VII.	Confined to bed.		
VIII.	Unconscious.		

59

distress states were selected as representing the full range of illness states. These states (IC, IID, VC, VIB, VIIB, VIID) were referred to as 'marker states'. All subjects carried out a magnitude estimation exercise in which they were asked initially to place the six marker states in rank order of severity. The subject was then presented with her first two cards, i.e. the least ill states and was asked 'How many times more ill is a person in state two as compared with state one?' In considering their response, the subjects were told to assume the following:

(a) The descriptions related to a young to middle-aged adult.
(b) All states have the same prognosis and could be cured if the patient is treated. If left untreated, the patient's condition would remain static until some other condition supervenes.

The question was then repeated using successive pairs of marker states (2 and 3, 3 and 4, 4 and 5, 5 and 6). The subjects were encouraged to take as much time as they required in order to complete this task. In making a judgement about the relative severity of the various marker states, subjects were asked to bear in mind a number of implications that might influence their decision. First, the ratio selected for two marker states would determine the distribution of NHS resources to those states. Second, the ratio defined a point at which subjects were indifferent between curing one patient in the more severe state, and curing a number of patients in the less severe state. The value for each ratio was multiplied by that for the succeeding ratio, for example, given ratios for the 6 markers (a, b . . . f) as follows:

a:b   1:3
b:c   1:6
c:d   1:12
d:e   1:4
e:f   1:5

Marker states would receive scores of:

a	b	c	d	e	f
1	3	18	216	864	4,320

The ranked marker states and their provisional scores provided a framework within which the remaining 23 states were ranked. Subjects were free to change the position of all states at any time. Once the ranking had been decided, the *scores* for all intermediate states were established. In particular, the subject was asked to assign a score of zero to the state to which he or she thought it reasonable to restore all patients. During this valuations task, subjects were again reminded that the value for any state could be modified.

At this point the subjects were asked to change the initial assumptions about prognosis, and to consider that the descriptions now applied to permanent states, none of which would be treated. Any changes to their valuations were noted. The final element in this procedure involved subjects locating death amongst the disability/distress states and placing a valuation on it.

As is often the case with such data, the distribution of scores was widely dispersed. Statistical analysis of these psychometric data revealed significant differences between medical and psychiatric patients, medical patients and doctors, medical nurses and doctors. Closest agreement was evident in the responses of patients and their nurses. No significant differences were detected in valuations when subjects were regrouped according to individual characteristics – including age, sex, social class, religion, and past history of illness (Rosser and Kind 1978). Doctors place relatively less emphasis on the importance of death in comparison with other states; their valuations resembled those of healthy volunteers and differed from those of patients and nurses. Doctors also placed more emphasis on the importance of subjective suffering.

The median valuations collected from Rosser's 70 subjects were originally published in a form which fixed the score for the healthy state IA as zero, but left all other states with unconstrained scores. This allowed a number of states to be regarded as worse than death (Kind and Rosser 1979). Subsequently these scores were transformed so that death received a score of 0 and 1A received a score of one. It is this latter scale (see Table 2) which has provided the valuations for use in current QALY applications.

The weights generated in Rosser's original work were never designed to be, or portrayed as being, representative of society as a whole. Furthermore the Rosser classification forms only one method of describing illness states. Many of the methodological questions encountered in measuring quality of life are currently being

Table 2 Transformed valuations for 29 health states

Disability	A	B	C	D
			Distress	
I	1.000	0.995	0.990	0.967
II	0.990	0.986	0.973	0.932
III	0.980	0.972	0.956	0.912
IV	0.964	0.956	0.942	0.870
V	0.946	0.935	0.900	0.700
VI	0.875	0.845	0.680	0.000
VII	0.677	0.564	0.000	−1.486
VIII	−1.028	—	—	—

Fixed points: Healthy = 1   Dead = 0

See: Kind, Rosser, and Williams (1982).

examined as part of a major research programme at the Centre for Health Economics at the University of York. The discussion in the remainder of this section takes a wide view of the measurement of the quality of life, including a description of alternative methodologies, and its use in areas other than health.

REFERENCES

Kaplan, R. M., Atkins, C. J., and Timms, R. (1984) 'Validity of a quality of well-being scale as an outcome measure in chronic destructive pulmonary disease', *Journal of Chronic Diseases* 37 (2):85–95.

Kind, P., Rosser, R., and Williams, A. (1982) 'Valuation of quality of life: some psychometric evidence', in M. W. Jones-Lee (ed.) *The Value of Life and Safety*, Leiden: North Holland, pp. 159–70.

Rosser, R. and Kind, P. (1978) 'A scale of valuations of states of illness: is there a social consensus?', *International Journal of Epidemiology* 7 (4):347–58.

Kind, P., and Rosser, R. (1979) 'Death and dying: scaling of death for health status indices', in B. Barker *et al.* (eds) *Lecture Notes on Medical Informatics*, Berlin: Springer-Verlag, 28–30.

Rosser, R. and Watts, V. C. (1972) 'The measurement of hospital output', *International Journal of Epidemiology* 1 (4):361–8.

Weinstein, M. C. and Stason, W. B. (1977) 'Foundations of cost-effectiveness analysis for health and medical practices', *New England Journal of Medicine* 296:716–21.

Weinstein, M.C. and Stason, W.B. (1985) 'Cost-effectiveness of interventions to prevent or treat coronary heart disease', *American Review of Public Health* 6:41–63.

Williams, A. (1985) 'Economics of coronary artery bypass grafting', *British Medical Journal* 291:326–9.

Chapter Four

ISSUES IN THE DESIGN AND CONSTRUCTION OF A QUALITY OF LIFE MEASURE

P. KIND

'Quality of life' has become the latest catchphrase to decorate the newspaper headlines and to enhance the impact of political debate. Its meaning is usually left to the reader's own imagination since it is seldom defined, instead being exemplified in terms of the context in which it is used, for example: personal security within the community, access to the performing arts, or the provision of decent housing. All these may indeed form part of the overall picture but they do not themselves uniquely characterize the concept quality of life, nor are they of direct relevance to those concerned with the commitment of health-care resources.

Clinicians, as well as Chief Constables, also refer to 'quality of life' in their research activities and in their day-to-day practice. Very often they mirror the confusion in meaning which attends its wider use. So far as this paper is concerned, the term 'quality of life' covers broadly those health-related aspects of life which are capable of being modified by the provision of health care.

The term 'measurement', in the physical sciences conveys the impression of a precise operation based on well-established procedures, carried out in controlled laboratory settings and producing results which are expressed in terms of standardized units of measure. This scenario contrasts markedly with the attempts of social scientists to develop measures of health-related quality of life (referred to here as QoL). Not only is the phenomenon under investigation defined in many different ways, but there is varying opinion as to how it might be represented, and on whether it could or should be quantified. As a consequence there have been a number of distinct and, hitherto, largely uncoordinated efforts to develop measures of QoL.

The richness of this research endeavour is of course encouraging, but this very diversity is seized upon by some critics who see the need to discredit quality of life measurement, so as to thereby indict its application in health economics and its role as an aid to decision-making in the NHS.

This paper describes some of the design issues involved in constructing measures of QoL and is intended to help regularize the debate on QoL measurement by providing a framework in which to assess the strengths and weaknesses of instruments, both new and old.

DESCRIPTION

In spite of the fragmented research effort in this field a common understanding of the problems of constructing QoL measures has emerged. In order to measure quality of life we need first to *describe* it, preferably in such a way that different levels/states can be identified.

A descriptive system is required in order to make the simplest form of measurement possible, that is to establish a relationship between a subject (patient) and some point or level on a quality of life continuum. Such a descriptive system might be based on a conceptual model which expresses the researcher's personal views of the relevant and measurable aspects of health or upon an existing definition, for example that of the WHO, expressed in terms of social, emotional, and physical well-being. No matter how the descriptive components of the indicator are specified, researchers are at this point effectively limiting the extent to which their instrument is practically capable of registering different aspects and levels of quality of life. Those elements which are not explicitly included in the descriptive system will not be fully represented and any subsequent efforts to weight the system will undervalue their contribution. This may be less of a problem where a fairly well-defined group of patients or a single disease process is involved, since the researchers are more likely to have an intimate knowledge of the condition and its impact on the patient. Where researchers adopt this 'top-down' approach and specify the elements of the descriptive system themselves, without reference to a wider set of judges, there can be no certainty that all *relevant* components have been included. Precisely what constitutes relevance, and who judges it are important considerations in themselves.

The problem of designing a comprehensive descriptive system may be tackled in another way, so as to partially overcome the difficulty of judging what should be incorporated in the descriptions – namely asking individuals to provide the material directly. Surveying the community, or a specific patient group, can yield large volumes of descriptive material about the effects of ill-health on usual functioning and quality of life. These data might be expressed in terms of statements made by the individual respondents about themselves, or in more general terms about the effects of ill-health on other people. This open-ended approach to constructing the descriptive base produces an almost endless stream of information, much of it being fairly idiosyncratic, especially where the respondent is given the opportunity to speak about their own, or their family's experiences of ill-health. Analysis of these data itself poses some awkward problems for the researcher. Faced with an abundance of data he/she has to find some way of organizing, refining, and reducing it so as to produce a viable set of descriptions, preferably one in which the use of language is simple, non-technical, and unambiguous, and which is compact enough to permit subsequent valuation. The processes involved in this 'bottom-up' approach are likely to be every bit as judgemental as those which characterize the prior specification of the 'top-down' strategy. Some of the researcher's ideas about how the descriptive material should be organized will inevitably influence the direction of the data analysis. Techniques such as multidimensional scaling or factor analysis which may produce statistically acceptable representations of the empirical data still require the researcher him or herself to make decisions about how the dimensions/factors are labelled or described.

VALUATION

Although simple forms of measurement are possible using a descriptive system alone, the usefulness of such a system can be significantly enhanced by the addition of a valuation or scoring system which *quantifies* different levels of quality of life, thus permitting the magnitude of changes in quality of life to be observed and measured. Introduction of a valuation system raises additional problems however, and two issues in particular will have to be considered: whose valuations should be sought, and how should these be derived? The case might be argued for selecting ill people, as a group who perhaps have the most acute awareness of the effects of ill-health. Similarly doctors and other health-care professionals might be represented as having a broader and more objective view of the relative severity of health states – as the 'experts', they too should be consulted. Individuals in good health might be thought of as being more detached from the influences of training or experience and therefore capable of giving a less biased set of responses. Ultimately, of course, since decisions have to be taken about the allocation and use of health care resources, it might be thought appropriate that any weights which are to form part of a QoL measure should originate with politicians and the government. The use of a single reference group for weighting a QoL indicator is to be avoided unless the weights are only to be applied in the specific context of a single disease or condition. Multiple reference groups provide much needed information about the variability in scores which may arise from different subject groups.

Whilst the construction of a soundly based scoring system is an important requirement in developing a useful indicator, not all researchers have been concerned with a detailed examination of the processes involved. In some instances the scoring system has been specified by researchers themselves on the basis of an arbitrary weighting of their own design. A slightly less crude means of generating a scoring system for a descriptive QoL indicator involves surveying a population sample to establish the frequencies with which different health states are encountered. These frequency data might then be converted into a simple numeric scale using one of a variety of models (e.g. Guttman). The scoring system might be so arranged that commonly occurring health states were given the highest weighting and the least common states, presumed to be the more serious, attracted lower weights.

SCALING TECHNIQUES

The analysis of attitudinal and subjective response data drawn from a variety of sources, has a long and honourable tradition (e.g. Thurstone 1927) which continues to the present day (e.g. Orth and Wegener 1983). Stevens (1966) distinguishes between three types of scaling procedure which have been used for measuring non-physical stimuli comparable to health states, for example the seriousness of crime (Sellin and Wolfgang 1964). *Magnitude estimation* is designed to elicit valuations directly from subjects. A single health state might be designated as a reference state by the experimenter and this would be assigned a unit value. The subject is asked to indicate the magnitude of the ratio between that reference state and other health states and to express this ratio as a number. If states B and C scored 4 and 8 respectively when compared to the reference state A (with its pre-assigned value of 1), then that subject's scale values for A, B, and C would be taken as 1, 0.25, and 0.125. The geometric mean or median scores for the experimental subject group should be used to represent the average valuations for each state. Where the rank order of states has been established prior to magnitude estimation then it is permissible to work with successive pairs of states, rather than continually making judgements with respect to the reference state.

Category rating, in one or other of its variants, forces subjects to classify states into one of a limited number of ordered categories. These categories are sometimes represented as being separated by equal intervals, although this is a difficult assumption to sustain. The typical rating scale will at least be bounded by descriptions of the end categories. Subjects are expected to sort the states into categories according to, say, their 'perceived seriousness'. The mean category score for each state can be calculated from the pooled experimental data. In its basic form this type of scaling, unlike magnitude estimation, does not support the examination of individual differences between subjects. Two variants of the procedure can assist in this. Rank ordering can be treated as a form of category rating in which the number of categories is equal to the number of health states. The mean rank sum based on the pooled responses can be used as scale values for the group as a whole and correlation coefficients can be used to examine the association between subject rankings. Similarly, graphical rating procedures can be used to capture valuations. Ratings can be expressed on a visual analogue scale (often a 10 cm line), on which subjects record the point at which they consider a state should be located. The end points of the line may be labelled by a description ('unimportant'; 'extremely serious') or by a numeric value (0; 100). The scores for each state are obtained by simply measuring the distance along the line that has been marked by the subject.

Paired comparisons methods require subjects to make judgements about pairs of states, essentially answering the question 'Is state A worse than state B?' No estimate is made of the magnitude of the relationship. Judgements about all pairs of states are required for the original model and this typically necessitates $n \times (n-1)/2$ judgements, although modifications to the procedure can circumvent this limitation where large numbers of states are involved. The analysis of paired comparisons data usually precludes the possibility of examining responses from individual subjects but measures of internal consistency are easily calculated and can be used to indicate the quality of the subjects' performance and the extent of any agreement amongst them.

The measurement level of any indicator should be carefully assessed in the course of its design and construction. Indicators which are published without proper evaluation of their measurement properties are likely to be limited in their usefulness and prone to misuse for purposes which they are intrinsically unable to support. In particular the arbitrary use of numbers to designate different levels within an indicator may lead to their spurious use as weights or valuations. Care should be exercised, too, in the selection of the statistical tests which are used to analyse observations based on these indicators. Most forms of statistical analysis can be applied to data from interval or ratio scales which give rise to quantitative measurements (the arithmetic mean can legitimately be computed as a measure of central tendency, for example). Nominal and ordinal scales produce data which are essentially qualitative in character and should be subjected to non-parametric statistical tests (the mode or median would be the appropriate measure of central tendency in this case). If the theory and practice of scaling methods appears to be an unduly complex area of study the reader will find some reassurance in Torgerson's standard reference work on the subject (Torgerson 1958).

SELECTING A SCALING METHOD

The selection of the procedure for eliciting or generating valuations from subjects is crucial in two respects. First, the scaling method which is adopted may require multiple ratings of health states and this can prove impractical for any but the smallest set of descriptive systems. Individual subjects may not be able to complete more than one set of ratings without fatigue and consequent degradation in the reliability of their responses. Larger, more complex descriptive systems can be partitioned so that a single subject is exposed to only one segment for the purposes of collecting repeated ratings. This in turn calls for correspondingly larger numbers of subjects, so that sufficient judgements can be obtained for statistical analysis. The approach, however, seriously limits the opportunity for examining individual differences between subjects. A similar limitation holds if the scaling method aggregates judgements made by individual subjects, as with the method of paired comparisons. The single subject's preference matrix in this instance cannot be analysed using Thurstone's original model (1927), although models which can cope with such data have been more recently described (Bradley and Terry 1952). Categorical scaling methods have similar deficiencies.

The second consideration in selecting the scaling procedure is the measurement properties of the resultant scale. As has already been observed, the use of number is no guarantee of any arithmetic properties whatsoever in the final instrument. Their association with health states in some circumstances merely serves as a convenient labelling device. Some procedures give rise to scales with well-recognized measurement properties, although these cannot be automatically assumed, especially where the scaling process has been inadequately implemented or where the statistical analysis has been incomplete. Computing the relevant goodness-of-fit statistic can be a useful safeguard against incautious optimism. Violations of the theoretical assumptions upon which a scaling method is based should be critically assessed. A clear example of this can be seen in respect of the Nottingham Health Profile (McKenna *et al.* 1981) which has been shown to be defective in the scaling of the sleep category (Kind 1982). Failure to attend to this detailed examination of the empirical data can only create additional problems in a research area already fraught with difficulty.

Since no standard measures exist against which the scoring systems of QoL indicators can be validated, there is continuing controversy about the relative superiority of the various scaling techniques which have been employed and about the scale values which they produce. Scale values arrived at by different experimental procedures may or may not be in agreement. The selection of both scaling method and the form of the descriptive material have been shown to influence raters' responses (Llewellyn-Thomas *et al.* 1984).

The different measurements of temperature on Fahrenheit and Centigrade scales can be simply resolved and observations on one scale may be transformed into corresponding values on the alternate scale. Measurement of quality of life has not yet reached the point where the relationship between different scales is so readily explained.

Both descriptive and quantitative forms of QoL measurement are becoming increasingly commonplace and accepted as desirable, if not necessary, components of evaluative studies. These efforts to expand the area in which QoL measurement is applied should not, however, mask some of the underlying methodological considerations which themselves remain open for further investigation. In examining the relative advantages of existing QoL instrumentation a series of questions ought to be addressed. These should examine the basis of the descriptive content of the instrument, its origins, mode of selection, refinement and simplification. Once this foundation material has been reviewed the measurement properties of the instrument should be critically assessed. The methods used to establish any scoring system should be the subject of an equally thorough examination. It should not be surprising if many putative QoL measures fail to satisfy these stringent tests since they represent ideal standards which may have to accommodate to the information needs of the real world. For those who are actively involved in the design and construction of new QoL measures, however, they constitute important areas of activity on a collective research agenda and as such need to be vigorously pursued.

REFERENCES

Bradly, R. A. and Terry, M. E. (1952) 'Rank analysis of incomplete block designs. The method of paired comparisons', *Biometrica* 39:324–45.

Kind, P. (1982) 'A comparison of two models for scaling health indicators', *International Journal of Epidemiology* 2:271–5.

Llewellyn-Thomas, H., Sutherland, H. *et al.* (1984) 'Describing health states', *Medical Care* 22:543.

McKenna, S. P., Hunt, S. M., and McEwen, J. (1981) 'Weighting the seriousness of perceived health problems using Thurstone's method of paired comparisons', *International Journal of Epidemiology* 10:93–7.

Orth, B. and Wegener, B. (1983) 'Scaling occupational prestige by magnitude estimation and category rating methods: a comparison with the sensory domain', *European Journal of Social Psychology* 13:417–31.

Sellin, T. and Wolfgang, M. E. (1964) *The Measurement of Delinquency*, New York: John Wiley.
Stevens, S. S. (1966) 'A metric for the social consensus', *Science* 151 (4 Feb.):530–41.
Thurstone, L. I. (1927) 'A law of comparative judgement', *Psychological Review* 34:273–86.
Torgerson, W. S. (1958) *Theory and Methods of Scaling*, New York: John Wiley.

Chapter Five

MULTIDIMENSIONAL REPRESENTATION OF DISABLEMENT
A qualitative approach[1]

MICHAEL HIRST

INTRODUCTION

Inasmuch as a quality of life concept is important for framing policies, evaluating programmes and making decisions, information on the set of conditions relevant to the concept is required. To aid understanding and interpretation, it is often necessary to summarize and display such information in a simpler and more accessible form. One approach aims to aggregate quality of life indicators into simple, global measures; the calculation of QALYs (quality adjusted life years), described above by Paul Kind, is an example. Another approach argues that human needs and welfare are multi-dimensional in essence, and therefore a multidimensional representation is required. This approach is adopted here; the aim is to organize data on one aspect of quality of life – disablement – in a comprehensive and analytically useful way.

Data on disablement describe and classify the experiences of people with disabilities and are required not only for policy making and service planning but also for decision making at the level of clinical and social work. However, there has been little debate about how representations of data on disablement might be constructed and interpreted (for an exception, see Williams 1979). Moreover, applications of conventional classification and scaling techniques have not been rigorously validated as representations of disablement (Duckworth 1983). Rather, attention has focused – rightly – on the meaning of disablement: on what information is required and on why information is being collected (Bury and Wood 1978; Walker 1980; Oliver 1987).

Nevertheless, the way disablement experiences are depicted can have important implications for policy and decision making, not least because the valuations or judgements often required by different methods are inherently political and not merely technical. It can also have implications for what data are required, how they are collected, and by whom. In this paper, it is argued that conventional methods are largely inappropriate and an alternative, structural approach to the representation of disablement is then outlined and evaluated.

DATA ON DISABLEMENT

Following Wood and Badley (1980), information on disablement can be characterized by two key properties:

(a) data on disablement describe individuals' subjective experience: such information is usually in the form of imprecise verbal descriptions.
(b) data on disablement are multidimensional; individuals usually describe many different aspects when interpreting their disablement experience.

The implication is that the methods used to construct representations of disablement should respect both the complexity and the qualitative nature of the information.

The relationship between a set of people with disabilities and a set of disablement experiences can be stored in a binary or logical array (Figure 5.1). The set of disablement descriptors may include medical definitions which stress individual defects and deficiencies, or it may encompass an economic perspective which focuses on vocational limitations. It may also encompass a socio-political perspective which views disablement as a product of the interaction between the individual, the physical environment, and society at large; in this case the descriptors might include environmental problems, social barriers, service provision, or policies which disable people with impairments. Moreover, the disablement descriptors could refer to houses, schools, workplaces, or localities for example, rather than to individuals. The precise categories and orderings included in a set of disablement experiences will of course vary according to purpose and should, ideally, be developed by the communities in question.

Figure 5.1 A binary array for storing the relations between *m* individuals and *n* disablement experiences

	Descriptors								
Case Number	Y_1	Y_2	Y_3	.	.	Y_j	.	.	Y_n
X_1						.			
X_2						.			
X_3						.			
.						.			
X_i	.	.	.	.	.	Z_{ij}	.	.	Z_{in}
.						.			
X_m						Z_{mj}			

$Z_{ij} = 1$ if the relation between X_i and Y_j is true; otherwise, $Z_{ij} = 0$

An equally important consideration for constructing this array is that the words used to describe disablement experiences should be at the same level of generality. This means for example, that a set of disabilities should not include walking, running, and climbing diffi-culties as well as locomotor problems since this term covers the other three. Sets of descriptors need, therefore, to be sorted into different degrees of generality according to common definitions; the interpretation of disablement experience is then carried out at what-ever level or levels are appropriate and useful. (For further dis-cussion of this idea of the hierarchy of terms and associated cover sets, see Atkin 1981.)

Entries in the array are denoted 1, meaning present or true, if an individual describes a particular disablement experience and 0 otherwise. Reading along a row of this array provides a profile or description of an individual in terms of his or her disablement experiences; reading down a column identifies those individuals who report the same disablement experience. Sometimes an ordinal relation may be established in which case a disablement experience is rated in terms of severity or intensity. Few disablement descriptors attain the level of measurement required for an interval or ratio scale and it is assumed that data on disablement will be measured at the nominal (binary) or ordinal level, that is, in discrete qualitative cate-gories. Whether the relation is binary or ordinal, it is important to stress that these data are not numerical quantities but verbal descriptions or labels. As a consequence, identical labels for different descriptors cannot be assumed equivalent and the data cannot be subject to arithmetical operations which assume quantitative measurement.

CONVENTIONAL APPROACHES TO REPRESENTATION

In a clinical or social work setting where the aim is to help the individual, a detailed assessment of needs and difficulties can be conveniently represented by a profile of scores on different dimensions of disablement. This could form a single row of the array described above. For the broader purposes of policy development, resource allocation, service planning, and evaluation however, the complexity of this approach creates difficulties. Comparisons between individuals or groups of individuals are required and there is a need to summarize and simplify information. Conventional approaches include summary or composite indices (Duckworth 1980), multidimensional scaling (Charlton, Patrick and Peach 1983), cluster analysis (Reid, Ballinger, and Heather 1978) and principal components analysis (Jarvis and Hey 1984), as well as specially derived indices of disablement (Rosser and Watts 1972; Humphreys *et al.* 1984). These methods seem inappropriate for three reasons:

(a) They require quantitative assumptions. Such techniques treat individuals as statistical entities and represent information on disablement experiences as if it were numerical data. Moreover, measures such as similarity coefficients, factor loadings, and group centroids are often arbitrarily determined by the choice of method.
(b) They involve loss of information. Conventional approaches use functional models which distort or destroy the essentially relational structure of individuals' disablement experience. As a consequence, any inherent complexity is often not reflected in the representation obtained and the original data, that is, individual profiles, cannot be recovered from the resulting factor scores, indices, or distance scales.[2]
(c) They require *a priori*, preference, or statistical weighting of each aspect of disablement and the trade-off between them. As far as is practicable, valuations should be accommodated after the data have been summarized, that is at the policy level.

Otherwise, the definition and description of disablement experiences will reflect the often hidden valuations which have entered as apparently technical judgements.

The rest of this paper describes a structural approach to the representation of disablement which overcomes these weaknesses. The most effective way of understanding the characteristics of this approach is through a specific example. The general qualities of the method can then be introduced and practical applications outlined.

Table 5.1   Incidence of severe impairment and disability in a sample of young people with spina bifida

| Case number | Impairments & disabilities | | | | | | | | | Key: |
	a	b	c	d	e	f	g	h	i	
1.	0	0	0	0	0	0	0	0	0	a. Incontinence
2.	1	1	0	0	0	0	0	0	0	b. Walking disability
3.	1	0	0	0	0	0	0	0	0	c. I.Q. < 85
4.	1	1	1	0	0	0	0	0	0	d. Abnormal appearance
5.	1	0	1	1	0	0	0	0	0	e. Epilepsy
6.	1	1	0	0	0	0	0	0	0	f. Manual disability
7.	1	1	1	0	0	0	0	0	0	g. Speaking disability
8.	1	1	0	0	0	0	0	0	0	h. Hearing disability
9.	1	1	0	0	0	0	0	0	0	i. Seeing disability
10.	0	1	0	1	0	0	0	0	0	
11.	1	1	1	0	0	0	0	0	0	1 = present
12.	1	1	1	1	0	1	0	0	0	0 = absent
13.	1	1	1	1	0	0	0	0	0	
14.	0	1	0	0	0	0	0	0	0	
15.	0	0	0	0	0	0	0	0	0	
16.	1	1	0	0	0	0	0	0	0	
17.	1	1	0	1	1	0	0	0	0	
18.	1	0	0	0	0	0	0	0	0	
19.	0	0	1	0	0	0	0	0	0	
20.	1	1	1	0	0	0	0	0	0	
21.	1	1	0	0	0	0	0	0	0	
22.	1	1	1	1	1	0	0	0	0	
23.	0	0	0	1	0	0	0	0	0	
24.	1	1	0	1	0	0	0	0	0	
25.	1	1	0	0	0	0	0	0	0	
26.	1	1	1	0	0	0	0	0	0	
27.	1	1	1	1	0	0	0	0	0	
28.	1	1	1	0	0	0	0	0	0	
29.	1	1	0	1	0	0	0	0	0	
30.	1	1	0	0	1	0	0	0	0	

Figure 3.2 Lattice representation of the information in Table 5.1

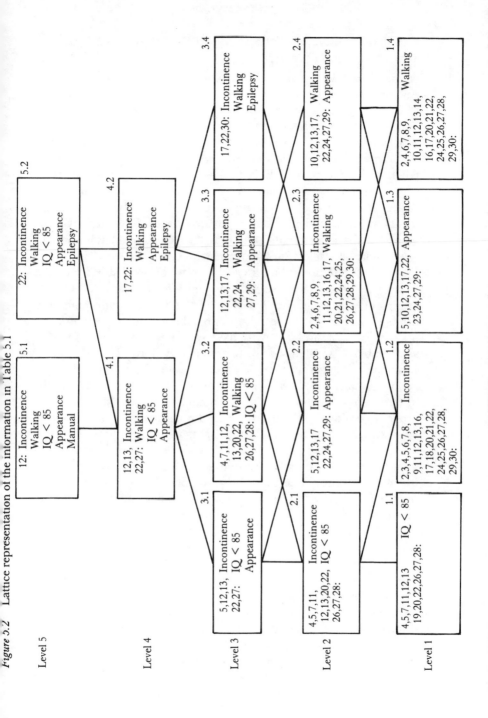

STRUCTURAL REPRESENTATION OF DISABLEMENT

Table 5.1 presents information on the functional limitations of 30 young people with spina bifida who formed part of a study by Anderson and Clarke (1982). The young people were aged 15 to 19 years and their day-to-day functioning was assessed using a modified form of the Pultibec system developed by Lindon (1963). This system incorporates a grading of severity for a range of functions likely to affect personal autonomy, social participation, educational potential, and employability. For simplicity, only nine functions were included here and the ratings of severity were dichotomized as severe or otherwise.[3] The question of distinguishing between impairments and disabilities was not pursued by Anderson and Clarke because their assessments predated the recommendations for an international classification (World Health Organization 1980).

A structural representation can be derived from Table 5.1 in two stages (Ho 1982; Macgill 1985). The array is first decomposed into groups of young people who display the same impairments and disabilities. For example, there are three young people (case numbers 17, 22, and 30) who have severe epilepsy, incontinence, and mobility problems and together they form a grouping or component. Altogether there are sixteen unique groupings of young people and functional limitations. Next these components are linked to form a lattice; to do this, components are placed in descending order according to the number of impairments and disabilities represented. Links between components at different levels are then made when the impairments and disabilities in a component are a subset of the components at the levels above and the young people in a component are a subset of the components at the levels below (Figure 5.2). For example, component 3.4 consisting of three young people with severe epilepsy, incontinence, and walking problems is linked 'upwards' to component 4.2 comprising two of the young people who also have abnormal appearance; it is also linked 'downwards' to component 2.3 which includes the three young people together with eighteen others who have severe incontinence and walking problems.

The lattice provides a complete classification of mutually shared impairments and disabilities by revealing all the inter-relationships between individuals and their disablement experiences. No arithmetical operations or valuations are imposed on the data and their qualitative nature is preserved. Moreover there is no loss of information: it is possible to reproduce the profile of impairments and disabilities experienced by each individual by finding the highest level at which that individual is placed in the lattice. For example, case number 10 is placed no higher than component 2.4: this young person therefore has two severe impairments and disabilities, walking problems and abnormal appearance. It is also possible to identify which individuals, and therefore how many, are alike in terms of their disablement experience and which of these experiences are found together. For example, ten young people have abnormal appearance (component 1.3) and twenty-three have severe walking problems (component 1.4), but only eight young people share both problems (component 2.4); and only seven young people have both these problems and severe incontinence (component 3.3). In this way it is possible to move up or down the lattice to examine any part of the structure whilst remaining aware of how it is embedded within the whole. Lastly, there is no redundancy or duplication in the lattice representation: the components comprise the minimum number necessary to avoid loss of information and those combinations which are contained within others are ignored. Thus three young people have severe epilepsy, but each has walking problems and incontinence as well (component 3.4), so epilepsy on its own does not appear as a separate component.

BACKCLOTH AND TRAFFIC

Following Atkin (1974, 1981), the pattern of relations depicted by the lattice can be thought of as a relatively stable backcloth. Like a theatrical stage set for a drama, this backcloth can then be conceived as allowing or forbidding certain activities or behaviours – what Atkin calls traffic. This backcloth/traffic distinction is akin to the more familiar one of pattern and process and suggests a potentially fruitful way of looking at disablement experiences. On a backcloth describing disablement, traffic could be extra living costs, receipt of services, employment and housing choices, claims for cash benefits, prognoses or other valuations, and so on. Changing the backcloth implies changing the pattern of relations between individuals and their experience of disablement, for example, by acquiring skills, using aids and appliances, adapting the environment, introducing anti-discrimination legislation, changing public attitudes, or as a result of recovery or deterioration. Such structural changes may support a different pattern of activities or traffic which may, in turn, lead to further change in the backcloth. The implication is that, although the form and content of disablement is relevant, not least to those with disabilities, it is the dynamics of traffic, and of backcloth and traffic changes, which give meaning to the experience of disablement. Focusing on the dynamic of disablement experiences can lead to a reconsideration of form and content and how they might be altered.

This perspective is as yet undeveloped, although a backcloth/ traffic distinction has been made in recent studies where a structural approach to the representation of disablement was adopted. In one study, the pattern of impairments and disabilities presented by 119 young people with cerebral palsy or spina bifida in Anderson and Clarke's study (1982) was represented by a lattice and two handicap scales assessing pyschological adjustment and quality of social life were conceived as traffic (Hirst 1989). The results showed that poor psychological adjustment and extreme social isolation were associated not so much with individual functional limitations as with particular configurations of impairments and disabilities. It seemed that social handicap was neither a necessary nor a direct consequence of any impairment or disability but arose generally from severe functional loss and was shaped by dependency on others, restricted choices, problems of physical access, and adverse reactions of others.

In another study, Richardson *et al.* (1984) investigated the use of residential and day services in relation to the pattern of disabilities displayed by young adults with a mental impairment. They found, for example, that there was no difference between those not receiving any service and those in long-term day or residential care in the frequency of behaviour disturbance alone; but those in long-term residential care more often had behaviour disorders in combination with other disabilities than those in day services or those not receiving services. The amounts received in social security benefits towards the extra costs of disablement have been examined in relation to the pattern of disabilities in a different sample of young people (Hirst 1986). It was found that those with disabilities arising from physical impairment received higher amounts on average than those with disabilities arising from mental impairment, the costs of which seemed to attract scant recognition in the social security system. Lastly, Hirst and Cooke (1988) investigated a paediatrician's assessment of overall severity of disablement in a sample of 10-year-old children. An attempt was made to identify combinations of disabilities which were good predictors of the paediatrician's assessment, illustrating one approach to mapping valuations onto a health-related backcloth.

CONCLUSION

A structural approach to the description and interpretation of disablement has been outlined. It reveals all the inter-relationships between individuals and their disablement experiences and provides an intuitively simple and robust representation for the purposes of classification. No information is lost in this representation. The approach therefore provides a bridge between those in a clinical or social work setting who need to represent individuals' experience of disablement, and policy makers, service planners, and others who need to make comparisons between individuals. A lattice representation of disablement could therefore form a basis for information retrieval and display by managers, professionals, and others who need to base their decision making on the way disablement experiences are related and combine. The lattice representation also provides a basis for investigating activities or processes which the disablement backcloth allows or constrains, and a starting point for investigating the implications of alternative valuations and interventions.

The approach is applicable to the representation of other aspects of health status and, indeed, to other quality of life categories. However, the lattice approach is not just another technique; defining a relational backcloth, identifying structural patterns, and exploring backcloth/traffic interdependency, provides a methodology for intrepreting and evaluating social structures which promises theoretical and practical insights.

NOTES

1   I am grateful to Michael Hearn for computer programming. The research was supported by the Department of Health and Social Security and the data were supplied by the ESRC archive. The author bears full responsibility for the analysis and interpretation reported here.
2   An exception is the Guttman scale, but this has limited application to data on disablement and assumes a cumulative pattern of scale items.

Information on individuals who do not conform to this assumption is lost. If the pattern of disablement experience is cumulative however, this would be revealed by the approach described here.

3 The approach requires a binary relation and ordinal relations can be transformed as here. It is possible of course to explore some or all of the binary relations contained in ordinal data according to purpose. The important point is that such choices are made explicit by the approach and their usefulness can then be scrutinized.

REFERENCES

Anderson, E. M. and Clarke, L. (1982) *Disability in Adolescence*, London: Methuen.

Atkin, R. H. (1974) *Mathematical Structures in Human Affairs*, London: Heinemann.

Atkin, R. H. (1981) *Multidimensional Man*, Harmondsworth: Penguin.

Bury, M. R. and Wood, P. H. N. (1978) 'Sociological perspectives in research on disablement', *International Rehabilitation Medicine* 1:24–32.

Charlton, J. R. H., Patrick, D. L., and Peach, H. (1983) 'Use of multivariate measures of disability in health surveys', *Journal of Epidemiology and Community Health* 37:296–304.

Duckworth, D. (1980) 'The measurement of disability by means of summed ADL indices', *International Rehabilitation Medicine* 2:194–8.

Duckworth, D. (1983) *The Classification and Measurement of Disablement*, London: HMSO.

Hirst, M. A. (1986) 'Disabilities, benefits, and disability benefits', *International Journal of Rehabilitation Research* 9:3–12.

Hirst, M. A. (1989) 'Patterns of impairment and disability related to social handicap in young people with cerebral palsy and spina bifida', *Journal of Biosocial Science* 21:1–12.

Hirst, M. A. and Cooke, K. (1988) 'Grading severity of childhood disablement: comparing survey measures with a paediatrician's assessment', *Child: Care, Health and Development* 14:111–26.

Ho, Y.-S. (1982) 'The planning process: structure of verbal descriptions, *Environment and Planning B* 9:397–420.

Humphreys, S., Lowe, K., and Blunden, R. (1984) 'The use of the degree of dependency scale for describing the characteristics of clients who are mentally handicapped', *British Journal of Mental Subnormality* 30:15–23.

Jarvis, S. and Hey, E. (1984) 'Measuring disability and handicap due to cerebral palsy', in F. Stanley and E. Alberman (eds) *The Epidemiology of the Cerebral Palsies*, Oxford: Blackwell.

Lindon, R. L. (1963) 'The Pultibec system for the medical assessment of handicapped children', *Developmental Medicine and Child Neurology* 5:125–45.

Macgill, S. M. (1985) 'Structural analysis of social data: a guide to Ho's Galois lattice approach and a partial respecification of Q-analysis', *Environment and Planning A* 17:1089–109.

Oliver, M. (1987) 'Re-defining disability: a challenge to research', *Research, Policy and Planning* 5:9–13.

Reid, A.H., Ballinger, B. R., and Heather, B.B. (1978) 'Behavioural syndromes identified by cluster analysis in a sample of 100 severely and profoundly retarded adults', *Psychological Medicine* 8:399–412.

Richardson, S. A., Koller, H., Katz, M., and McLaren, J. (1984) 'Patterns of disability in a mentally retarded population between ages 16 and 22 years', in J. M. Berg and J. M. de Jong (eds) *Perspectives and Progress in Mental Retardation, vol. II, Biomedical Aspects*, Baltimore: University Park Press.

Rosser, R. M. and Watts, V. C. (1972) 'The measurement of hospital output', *International Journal of Epidemiology* 1:361–8.

Walker, A. (1980) 'The social origins of impairment, disability and handicap', *Medicine in Society* 6:18–26.

Williams, R. G. A. (1979) 'Theories and measurement in disability', *Epidemiology and Community Health* 33:32–47.

Wood, P. H. N. and Badley, E. M. (1980) *People with Disabilities: Towards Acquiring Information which Reflects more Sensitively Their Problems and Needs.* New York: World Rehabilitation Fund.

World Health Organization (1980) *International Classification of Impairments, Disabilities, and Handicaps*, Geneva: World Health Organization.

Chapter Six

THE SCOPE AND LIMITATIONS OF QALY MEASURES

GRAHAM LOOMES and LYNDA McKENZIE

INTRODUCTION

The increasing interest in Quality Adjusted Life Years (QALYs) as an aid to health care decision making is a reflection of the growing awareness that health care choices frequently entail – either directly or indirectly – some trade-off between length of life and quality of life.

This paper discusses the validity of QALY methodology as advocated for use in two separate contexts: where choices have to be made between different possible forms of treatment[1] for the *same* individual; and in situations where a choice must be made between alternative ways of allocating limited resources among diverse health care activities.

The North American approach to QALY measurement is founded on decision analytic techniques (see Raiffa 1968), based on the conventional economic theory of individual choice under uncertainty, 'expected utility theory'. This theory, formalized by von Neumann and Morgenstern in the mid 1940s, was adopted only recently by the medical profession as a means of facilitating clinical decision making in a way that takes into account the subjective values and preferences of individual patients concerning both the outcomes of care and the inherent riskiness of the decision. While this 'individual' utility based model has also been applied to resource allocation choice problems, another type of QALY measure which has received considerable attention in Britain was specifically developed for decision making at the aggregate or policy level. We examine each of these approaches in terms of their central assumptions and validity in the light of both clinical and non-clinical evidence.

84

QALYS AND INDIVIDUAL UTILITY FUNCTIONS

The basic notion behind the QALY concept is that an individual who is faced with the prospect of living Y years at less than full health may be able to equate this to the prospect of living X years (where $X < Y$) at full health.

The idea then is that if any number of profiles of survival duration in a whole range of health states can be converted to their respective 'full health life years' equivalents, such QALY measures may be used as a decision aid in cases where different therapeutic options may produce quite diverse combinations of length and quality of life.

Moreover, if it is the case that, all other things being equal, individuals will choose options which offer more QALYs in preference to those which offer less, the argument is that it should be possible to locate QALYs in some more general utility model. Miyamoto and Eraker (1985), developing the work of Pliskin, Shepard, and Weinstein (1980), have considered the relationship between QALYs and a bivariate utility function[2] specified as follows in Equation (1):

$$U(Y, Q) = bY^r H(Q)$$

where it is assumed that an individual will choose between alternatives so as to maximize utility, U, which depends on survival duration, Y, and health status, Q.

The parameter r represents the patient's risk attitude towards gambles involving survival duration, and $H(Q)$ measures the utility of survival in health state Q (where Q is normally less than full health) as a proportion of the utility of survival in excellent health. The parameter b is a scaling constant chosen so that the utility indices lie in some convenient range (say, 0–100).

Clearly if $b = 1$ and $r = 1$, (the latter indicating 'risk neutrality' with respect to survival duration), utility is simply given as expected length of life multiplied by a factor measuring the utility of survival duration in a particular health state relative to the utility of survival in excellent health. However, even if r is not equal to 1, utilities and QALYs correspond as long as $H(Q) = (X/Y)^r$.

Of course, the specification in Equation (1) is only one of many forms that a bivariate utility function could take. The QALY model is therefore a special case, and involves certain fairly severe restric-

85

tions. We now examine those restrictions more closely, and consider the relevant evidence.

Constant proportional time trade-off

One restriction involves the assumption of a constant proportional trade-off between length of life and health status. This entails an individual being prepared to 'sacrifice' some *constant proportion* of their remaining years of life in order to achieve a given improvement in their health status, irrespective of the absolute number of years that remain. So, for example, an individual who regards 12 years in excellent health as equivalent to 15 years in their current state of health is assumed to regard 4 years of excellent health as equivalent to 5 years in their current health state, and so on.

However, there are reasons, both empirical and theoretical, for doubting the validity of this assumption. A study by McNeil *et al.* (1981) suggested that individuals were only willing to trade longevity for an improvement in health status when the absolute length of time to be spent with a less than perfect level of speech was greater than five years. That is, as Y falls towards 5, X/Y tends to rise towards 1.0.

Miyamoto and Eraker acknowledged these findings, but defended the QALY model on the grounds that the results may be rather specific to treatment choice for laryngeal cancer and that, even if the QALY model is not infallible, it serves a useful purpose as a heuristic approach to incorporating patients' preferences in clinical decisions.

Such arguments are, however, weakened in view of additional conflicting evidence. Sackett and Torrance (1978) found that the values which people placed on various health states differed significantly with the duration of the states. And in their study, Sutherland *et al.* (1982) discussed the concept of a 'maximal endurable time', which they introduced to represent the length of time beyond which individual preferences over alternative health scenarios changed dramatically relative to preferences involving shorter periods of time in the same health state.

Pliskin, Shepard, and Weinstein (1980) reported 30 pairs of time trade-off responses from 10 subjects presented with (hypothetical) questions concerning the relief of different levels of anginal pain. Of these, only 9 pairs of responses were strictly consistent with the constant proportional time trade-off assumption, and five of these involved zero sacrifice of longevity. In other words, out of 25 pairs of responses from individuals who were prepared to sacrifice some length of life for relief of anginal pain, only 4 were consistent with the assumption.

Presumably Miyamoto and Eraker also have data on this question. In order to estimate $H(Q)$, they put two time trade-off questions to each of 46 patients suffering from symptomatic coronary artery disease, one question using $Y = 12$, the other using $Y = 25$. Unfortunately, they did not report the extent to which the answers do or do not correspond with the assumption, although they did say that 'the reliability of the estimates and the validity of the assumed model have not been determined' (1985:205). They urged further investigation to see 'whether model violations are sufficiently widespread and of large enough magnitude to preclude its application' (1985:208). Certainly, on the basis of the limited, but rather unfavourable, evidence so far concerning the constant proportional time trade-off assumption, there is reason to be cautious.

A further reason to be cautious is that, as it stands, the model makes no *explicit* allowance for time preference. In its most general form, the notion of time preference is that the value an individual places on an event may vary with the timing of that event. For example, it is often assumed that individuals prefer present consumption of a commodity to future consumption of that same commodity, so that the utility of future consumption is discounted for time.

This raises the question of whether the 'consumption of life' might be regarded in the same way, i.e. whether more distant periods in a given health state might be valued differently from periods now and in the near future. If this were the case, it would tend to undermine the constant proportional time trade-off assumption. For example, if a geometrically declining series of weights were attached to future periods, it is straightforward to show[3] that for any given health state rated lower than excellent health, the *proportion* of Y that individuals would be prepared to sacrifice to achieve excellent health will increase as Y increases. This appears to be consistent with some of the evidence cited above, such as that reported by McNeil *et al.* (1981) although the study by Buxton *et al.* (1986), which involved a range of health states, suggests that the pattern may be more complex.

87

Other factors, when combined with 'pure' time preference, may help to explain these more complex patterns of valuation of future periods, which may be associated with 'thresholds' in a person's life-cycle where sharp changes may occur in the way in which valuations are made over present and future events. For example, it is conceivable that a young single adult may place a lower weight on good health now than on good health a few years ahead when he or she may be raising a young family; the weight placed on good health in years beyond that, when the children have grown up, may then fall; but may rise again for the years immediately following retirement, when the individual may hope to take advantage of greater leisure time opportunities. Some indications of these kinds of considerations were detected by Pliskin, Shepard, and Weinstein (1980:218–19). A more recent study, reported in Williams (1988), provided further relevant evidence on a larger scale. A sample of 377 individuals were asked to consider a set of twelve 'life-stages', and to choose and rank the three where they thought it was most important for an individual to be in full health. Although such a study gives only limited information about *strength* of preference, it suggests that very many people may value certain later stages of life more highly than some earlier stages, and therefore adds to the doubts already expressed about the validity of the constant proportional time trade-off assumption.

Independence and constancy of risk attitude to survival duration

Most health care alternatives involve some degree of risk and uncertainty, and therefore individuals' attitudes to risk are liable to affect the choices they make between different alternatives. We have seen that in Equation (1), risk attitude towards uncertain duration of survival is represented by the parameter r. The QALY utility model requires that the value of r for any individual should be independent of health state, and that the individual's utility function should exhibit constant proportional risk attitude.

To see the significance of this, consider the case where $b = 1$, where $H(Q) = h$, and where the individual is faced with a prospect involving a probability of p of living for Y_1 years in that health state, and a probability of $1-p$ of living for Y_2 years in the same health state. Let us write this prospect as $(Y_1 h, p; Y_2 h, 1-p)$.

Depending on the individual's attitude to risk, there will be some length of life between Y_1 and Y_2 denoted Y_c, such that the individual will be indifferent between the certainty of living Y_c years in the particular health state, and the risky prospect. Formally (Equation (2)):

$$(Y_c h, 1) \sim (Y_1 h, p; Y_2 h, 1-p)$$

The independence of risk attitude from health status requires that if the individual were faced with a prospect involving the same probability distribution of lengths of life, but in a different health state where $H(Q) = \alpha h$, the certainty equivalent length of life would be unaffected, so that (Equation (3)):

$$(Y_c \alpha h, 1) \sim (Y_1 \alpha h, p; Y_2 \alpha h, 1-p)$$

Constant proportional risk attitude with respect to survival duration requires that if, instead of changing the health state, we were to change both Y_1 and Y_2 to αY_1 and αY_2 respectively, we should change the certainty equivalent by the same factor, so that (Equation (4)):

$$(\alpha Y_c h, 1) \sim (\alpha Y_1 h, p; \alpha Y_2 h, 1-p)$$

The equivalence of the left hand sides of Equations (3) and (4) is, of course, fundamental to the QALY utility model. However, the direct evidence about the assumption of constant proportional risk attitude in uncertain health care choices is rather scant. Pliskin, Shepard, and Weinstein based their estimates of r on just one question. Miyamoto and Eraker asked two questions, one assuming no angina, the other assuming angina was present. Their estimate of r was the arithmetic mean of the values of r derived from the two questions, but they did not show any analysis which might indicate the extent or direction of any differences in individuals' responses to these questions.

In the absence of more direct evidence, we might consider some indirect evidence from the substantial body of empirical research into risky prospects involving wealth. Although it will not necessarily be the case that behaviour towards financial risks is echoed in the way people handle risks involving health or longevity, we shall see that there are at least some known parallels.

The literature concerning estimates of the characteristics of utility functions, and tests of the basic assumptions underlying such functions, is large and growing. Three relatively recent surveys (Schoemaker 1982; Machina 1983; Farquhar 1984) give a good indication of the scope and scale of the work done and the problems encountered.

For example, there is a great deal of evidence, dating back to Friedman and Savage (1948) and occurring in many other forms since, to suggest that an individual's attitude to risk cannot be represented, as in Equation (1), by a constant value of r: indeed, the same individual may systematically exhibit both risk aversion and risk seeking, and do so both in the domain of gains and of losses. If this kind of behaviour were to be translated more generally into health care decisions, it would clearly undermine the QALY assumption of constant proportional risk attitude.

A more general class of observations constitute the 'utility evaluation effect' (See Machina 1983:72–6 and Farquhar 1984: Sections 5–7 for details). The essential point here is that different procedures for eliciting preferences, or even different variants of the same procedures, produce systematically different estimates of utilities for the same sets of outcomes. This seems to be very similar to what Llewellyn-Thomas *et al.* (1984) found when using different approaches to obtain values for health states. In particular, they found that using a von Neumann-Morgernstern standard gamble method, and using a category rating approach, generated substantial and systematic differences in the scores and preference orderings from the same subjects for the same set of health states. Similar results were also reported in a study using three different utility measurement techniques: Bombardier *et al.* (1982) found that different utility scores for the same set of health state scenarios were derived using the standard gamble method of certainty equivalence compared with either the time trade-off or visual analogue (category rating) techniques. They attribute the systematically higher utility scores to a gambling effect, which they distinguish from risk aversion, whereby people place a higher value on a health state when it is offered as a certain option in an uncertain choice problem than when no options are specified as probabilistic.

One example of another potentially serious practical and theoretical difficulty is the 'framing effect'. Kahneman and Tversky

(1979) presented evidence that individuals' stated preferences between alternatives could be substantially affected by the way in which the alternatives were 'framed': in particular, if a pair of prospects were presented in terms of probabilities of gains, the pattern of choice was very different from when the (formally identical) pair of prospects were couched in terms of losses.

Kahneman and Tversky observed a similar pattern for (hypothetical) problems involving human life as for problems involving sums of money. McNeil *et al.* (1982) provided parallel results when they observed many of the patients in their study to have substantially different preferences over surgical as opposed to non-surgical treatment options according to whether the outcomes of treatment were described in terms of probabilities of living or probabilities of dying.

Clearly, these latter studies go beyond the issue of whether we can reasonably assume constant proportional risk attitude, and raise questions about whether we can get *any* reliable estimate of individuals' utility functions. This problem is compounded by other doubts about the descriptive validity of the independence assumption.

Besides the role that independence plays in the QALY model, it is in general the axiom that does much of the work in utility evaluation, since it postulates that the utility assigned to any particular outcome in a prospect is independent of the nature and probability of the other possible outcomes, or the other prospects in the set from which the choice is being made. The range, scale, and persistence of patterns of violation of the independence axiom in non-medical decisions should, at the very least, alert researchers who are using an independence assumption in medical decision making to the need to check the robustness of that assumption in the context in which they are working.

An important consideration in many health care decisions can of course be the possibility of immediate death – during or shortly after surgery, for example. As such, the decision may be thought of in terms of at least three possible outcomes from a choice between two forms of treatment, surgery and medical management. It is feasible to include the possibility of surgical mortality in the QALY approach by allowing Y to be zero.

Neither Pliskin *et al.* nor Miyamoto and Eraker included the possibility of immediate death in their analysis. However, Weinstein *et al.* (1977) found that individuals' choices between surgical (CABG) and non-surgical treatment could be influenced radically by the chance of surgical mortality. Additional evidence can be found in the results of work by Llewellyn-Thomas *et al.* (1982) who conclude that the standard gamble method is itself internally inconsistent on the basis that individuals in their experiments exhibited consistently different preference orderings over a range of alternative health states according to whether or not the choice between health state prospects included death as a possible outcome.

However, even in cases which do not involve the risk of immediate death, there is a more general problem relating to the treatment of time. Evidence that individuals can exhibit labile preferences was reported by Christensen-Szalanksi (1984) who found that women's preferences concerning choice of childbirth service changed over time both during pregnancy and post-natally.

Machina (1983:92) suggests that 'the "induced" or derived preferences of agents in situations of delayed risk . . . will typically not satisfy the independence axiom even if underlying individual preferences do'. Since many important health care decisions involve a considerable temporal element, including perhaps substantial changes in life expectancy and the distribution of the probability of death, the application of conventional expected utility analysis may simply be inappropriate or, at best, may require substantial modification.

This leads on to the final problem raised in this section, which concerns the use of the 'certainty equivalent' notion. It may be reasonable to ask people to consider the value of the certainty of a particular sum of money and compare it with some risky monetary prospect. But it seems altogether less plausible to ask for the value of the certainty of X years of life, presumably followed by the certainty of death at the end of those X years. Leaving aside the issue of whether people really would prefer to know the length of their life and the date of their death with certainty, it is a prospect which simply cannot be delivered, and which probably cannot be accurately imagined and evaluated in the way that (perhaps) a certain sum of money might be.

If the response to this argument is that it is taking the notion of certainty equivalent too literally, and that what the certainty equivalent method is doing is simply providing a unidimensional yardstick by means of which people can express their preference orderings over more realistic multidimensional prospects, then the evidence from non-medical sources contains a further warning, in the form of the preference reversal phenomenon.

This phenomenon occurs when an individual, asked to choose between two risky prospects, A and B, chooses A; but when asked to place separate certainty equivalent valuations on each of them, places a higher value on B. As Slovic and Lichtenstein (1983:596) have pointed out, this phenomenon is both predictable and persistent, occurring even in studies 'motivated by a healthy skepticism of the phenomenon and a belief that, examined under proper conditions, it might disappear'. If certainty equivalents of risky prospects involving sums of money well within people's normal experience are unreliable guides to preferences between those prospects, it is hard to be confident that valuations of risky prospects involving states of health outside people's normal experience, and expressed in terms of certain lifespans, are likely to be any more reliable.

QALYs IN INDIVIDUAL AND SOCIAL DECISION MAKING

Many of the most active proponents of decision analysis are, of course, well aware of the difficulties. For example, in giving the Ninth Annual Lecture of the Geneva Association, Weinstein (1986) devotes the final section of his paper to discussing some of the 'limits and challenges'. He concludes as follows:

> This challenge, then, is to understand more about what patients, and potential patients, value about health care. It is clearly naive to assume that patients wish to maximize quality-adjusted life expectancy. But what do they wish to maximize? The more we learn about this question, the more acceptable will be the prescriptive models that seek to guide allocations of medical resources.

> The final challenge is related to the incentives facing health-care decision makers to allocate resources. Every health-care system needs to consider how to transfer the societal objective of maximizing health-related utility within global resource limits into a system of decentralized incentives for individual providers and institutions. With such incentives in place, decision analysis

and cost-effectiveness analysis will become important
management tools at all levels of health care.

(Weinstein 1986:214)

This conclusion expresses very well the dilemma facing researchers. QALY measures based on conventional expected utility theory
are known to be descriptively inadequate; yet they are related to an
axiomatic base which has considerable normative appeal, and they
appear to be at least as valid as simple life expectancy measures, or
even cruder and more arbitrary measures such as five-year survival
rates. Given that decisions have to be made, and cannot be post-
poned until researchers have perfected the decision tools, the use of
QALYs at their present stage of development may be defended as
being no worse than any alternative measure, and offering the
prospect of improvement.

It is tempting to think of QALYs rather like some innovative
surgical procedure or new pharmaceutical compound which is not
yet proven, but is thought to be worthy of clinical trial. The danger
is that, in making out the case for QALYs to be evaluated, sufficient
enthusiasm and belief in their superiority may lead them to be
widely adopted before they have been appraised with the rigour of a
clinical trial.

An indication of the possible danger is the apparently rather
uncritical way in which it is suggested that individual utility-based
QALYs can be used to generate measures of cost-effectiveness which
may then serve as a guide when setting health care priorities for
social decision making.

Implicit in Weinstein's approach, and in that of others such as
Torrance et al. (1982), seems to be the view that the values to be used
in social decision making should be some aggregate of individuals'
values. But this is not the only possible view: for example, the socio-
political system may designate certain people to make decisions on
society's behalf, and the values these decision makers use may not
be some aggregate of individuals' values, but may reflect some other
notion of what represents society's overall best interests.

So the use of individuals' valuations as the legitimate source of
values for social decisions is itself a value judgement. But even if we
accept that judgement, and even if the utility indices derived were
thought to be valid representations of individuals' preferences, it is

94

still necessary to invoke some extra principle of inter-personal comparability in order to allow aggregation across individuals. Frequently this is done by assigning a value of 1.0 to 'good health' and a value of 0 to death for all individuals, and then taking the arithmetic mean of the utility scores derived on this basis. According to Torrance: 'The central basis for this method is that the difference in utility between being dead and being healthy is set equal across people. In this way the method is egalitarian within the health domain; that is, each individual's health is counted equally' (1986:17).

Williams (1988) makes a similar judgement, but uses a rather different method of obtaining valuations of other health states. His starting point is the need for any society with scarce resources to set health care priorities, and his objective is to produce a global index capable of measuring benefits from a wide variety of interventions on a common scale (which he also calls QALYs). However, rather than use standard gamble techniques, he adopts Rosser and Kind's (1978) Classification of Illness States and its associated valuation matrix as the closest approximation currently available to the kind of instrument he requires.

Rosser and Kind (1978) describe how this valuation matrix was generated, and discuss its properties. The methodology is consistent with a ratio scale, although they are careful to state that 'extensive further work will be necessary to verify such a claim. . . . Until such further evidence is available, no substantial claims can be made as to the ratio property of this scale.'

Using the mean[4] values estimated by Rosser and Kind (1978), a number of illustrative cost-per-QALY calculations have been made – see, for example, Williams (1985, 1988) and Gudex (1986).

However, if the use of a (putative) ratio scale is regarded as an advantage for this approach *vis-à-vis* the von Neumann-Morgenstern utility-based QALY, there are other respects in which it appears to be relatively disadvantaged, and some in which both approaches seem to face various kinds of difficulties.

Some of the difficulties *may* be amenable to further research: at the very least, they require further thought and investigation. For example, the extent to which measures based on aggregating individual valuations neglect (or double count) externalities; whether and in what way discounting future years – or allowing for the possibility that some later years may be valued more highly than some earlier ones – can or should be incorporated and the extent to which using average measures of the quality of various states may lead to welfare loss by neglecting valuations at the margin.

Another issue requiring further research concerns what may be thought of as the analogue of the independence axiom for the Rosser–Kind–Williams approach: namely, whether the value placed on an illness state is independent of the time spent in that state, and whether the QALY equivalent for any profile of an individual's progress up and/or down through a succession of health states can be calculated simply by multiplying the time spent in each state by its quality-adjustment factor, and summing. Since the differences in outcomes which we are trying to measure typically take the form of differences in these time profiles, the independence assumption is clearly a crucial one to examine.

One reason for suspecting that the value attached to any particular time profile of health states cannot be simply decomposed into a number of independently valued segments is that the value which people place on their state of health at any point in time may depend not only on how disabled and distressed they feel at that moment, but may also be influenced by their perception of how their present health state will affect their future health. This is likely to lead to diverse values for chronic and acute forms of illness; an individual who experiences several months of moderate discomfort as part of a treatment which he expects to result in improvements may place a rather different value on that experience compared with an individual for whom the same period in the same state of discomfort is seen as a phase in a degenerative illness, with a much lower expectation of recovery; similarly, different values may be placed on health states according to whether or not the alleviation of distress/ disability is only short-lived with a subsequent return to a more chronic state.

This brings us to what is potentially the major disadvantage of the Williams approach relative to the von Neumann–Morgenstern utility-based approach, namely, its neglect of (or, at best, implicit natural assumption about) attitudes to risk and uncertainty. Rosser and Kind's valuations were obtained by asking people to compare the certainty of one state with the certainty of another. When applying these valuations to a risky prospect – such as coronary artery bypass grafting – Williams (1985) takes the values of the three broad outcomes (improvement, no improvement, peri-operative death) and multiplies them by their respective (objective) probabilities. This is only justified, of course, if individuals are risk neutral, or if a judgement is made that their attitudes to risk are to be disregarded.

However, if the dimensions chosen to form the basis of valuation are selected because of their importance to people's perceptions of what affects their quality of life – and this is the justification for selecting 'disability' and 'distress' as the dimensions of the Rosser–Kind matrix – then there is no case for disregarding risk and uncertainty or assuming risk neutrality, since we have plentiful evidence from clinical and non-clinical studies that these factors have a substantial non-neutral impact on valuation and choice – especially, as we saw earlier, when at least one of the alternatives involves some risk of immediate death.

Moreover, the difficulty is not confined to some cases where the outcomes of the alternative interventions are uncertain. Suppose we are asked to rank two interventions, A and B, whose effects are known with certainty: A generates an extra 3 QALYs for each person treated, while B generates 1 QALY per person treated. If A costs only twice as much as B per treatment, the cost-per-QALY calculation clearly favours A. But if the lower cost of B allows twice as many treatments to be provided, thereby increasing the probability of receiving this treatment, it is quite conceivable that the majority of a population might prefer the prospect which offers each of them as individuals a larger probability of a smaller QALY gain to the prospect of a smaller probability of a larger benefit, and might be willing to pay a kind of 'risk premium' by choosing the prospect which, in QALY terms, offers a lower expected value. Clearly, then, using QALY measures which effectively assume risk neutrality may lead to a quite different allocation of resources from the one which a majority of individuals might prefer.

The above example supposes that the majority of the population is risk averse. In fact, as noted earlier, there is evidence that many individuals simultaneously exhibit a mixture of risk aversion and risk seeking. In health care terms, this latter attitude may be consistent with a demand for some treatments which do poorly by the cost-per-QALY criterion, but which may be perceived to offer dramatic benefits for at least some of those treated. The reason for this is that QALYs are evaluated *ex post*, but if an element of 'insurance' is included, then *ex ante* values could be higher. Examples may include heart and liver transplants, and coronary and neonatal intensive care units: there is a very small probability that individuals will need and receive these treatments, although if they do, the benefits may be very considerable; and even predominantly risk averse individuals may want to include some items such as these in their 'portfolio of health care investments' in much the same way as Friedman and Savage (1948) observed that individuals who took out insurance were also willing to buy low-probability large-prize lottery tickets.

Of course, it might be argued that people may wish to have resources devoted to such things as intensive care units because they overestimate either the benefits offered, or the probability of needing such facilities. This points to a further problem: if individuals have poor perceptions about the probabilities of illness and/or the benefits associated with different treatments, might they not also have poor perceptions about the quality of life in health states with which they are unfamiliar?

Uncertainty about the value of other states of health may be a significant difficulty, especially if it results in substantial and systematic differences between *ex ante* and *ex post* valuations. For example, a number of those people interviewed for the Rosser and Kind (1978) study said that they regarded certain states as being as bad, or worse, than death. These kinds of statements have been recorded in other studies, e.g. the survey reported by Jones-Lee *et al.* (1985) where a majority of respondents said that they considered certain outcomes (of transport accidents) to be at least as bad as death. And yet it appears that when people are actually experiencing these states, many of them do *not* regard their lives as valueless, or as having negative value.

It is important to know more, not only about the size and extent of differences between *ex ante* and *ex post* valuations, but also about the reason(s) *why* such differences occur. One reaction to any systematic disparities may be to say that some judgement should be made to use one set of values or the other, but that this judgement is not for economists to make. However, that may depend on the reason(s) for the disparities.

One possible explanation for the disparities is that when their health state changes, people adjust their lives in ways which reduce the extent of the real loss compared with what they might have expected. The argument here is that moving to a poorer health state reduces the range of activities available to an individual and/or the amount of utility derived from those activities, but is unlikely to do so to exactly the same extent for all categories of activities: hence individuals change the balance of activities, substituting those which are still feasible for those which are no longer feasible, and/or those where the utility has been least diminished for those where the reduction has been sharpest.

A similar kind of argument may be applied to reductions in life expectancy. Reducing the expected length of remaining life by x per cent will not necessarily reduce the value of remaining life by x per cent, even if individuals expect to be in the same health state for nearly all of that remaining period: one reason is that individuals may reorganize their life-plans to make the best of their changed expectations, and this reorganization may result in an overall loss which is less than x per cent.

The significance of the previous two paragraphs is to suggest the possibility that since individuals can adapt and rearrange their lives (within limits, of course), and since their health state is not the sole and immutable determinant of what gives value and quality to their lives, even a ratio scale of illness states is not an adequate proxy for quality of life; and, more worryingly, *may* be liable to *systematically* misrepresent the relative values of different outcomes.

CONCLUSION

It may seem that the general tone of this paper has been somewhat negative, cataloguing the drawbacks and difficulties associated with QALYs, but neglecting to give due weight to their superiority compared with other measures currently being used, and failing to offer any better alternative.

However, is it certainly not our intention to be destructive. Quite the opposite: the purpose of this paper has been to try to draw together a number of the practical and theoretical problems that have arisen at various times in different studies, in order to focus attention on the broad issues that require further discussion and research. For if it is true that, even with all the difficulties that remain, QALYs represent a considerable step forward for individual and social decision making in the field of health care, how much more progress might be achieved if we can address, and perhaps resolve, some of the more serious of those remaining difficulties.

It is of course possible that in the process of this endeavour we may come to the conclusion that there are very considerable limitations to the QALY approaches – limitations too fundamental to be overcome simply by developing more sophisticated techniques for eliciting and estimating preferences and valuations. Weinstein (1986:213) acknowledged this possibility: 'More radical solutions may involve rejecting the expected utility model as a prescriptive basis for action, given that it does not seem to perform well descriptively.' If this does turn out to be the eventual conclusion, then the sooner we move in that direction the better; and it seems likely that the best way of evaluating this possibility is to confront the various shortcomings in an open-minded way to try to determine the nature and extent of the 'adverse side-effects' associated with QALYs, compared with the benefits they may bring. For the use of QALYs in health care decision making has at least as much potential for welfare gain or loss as any new pharmaceutical compound or surgical procedure, and we should be at least as stringent in our evaluation of QALYs as we would wish to be when appraising any other innovation.

NOTES

1 The term 'treatment' should be interpreted very broadly, to include a wide spectrum of health care interventions ranging from education and prevention to long-term care for elderly or terminally ill people.
2 This is an extension of the univariate utility function based on axioms proposed originally by von Neumann and Morgenstern (1947). A clear exposition of the notion of bivariate utility functions, illustrated with a medical example, can be found in Raiffa (1968).
3 Let the current year be denoted y_0, the next year be y_1, and so on. To focus attention on the impact of time preference let $b, r = 1$. Suppose there is a discounting factor, d (where $d < 1$), such that y_i is discounted by a factor d^i. Then Y years at some health state Q less than full health can be discounted to a 'present value' PV:

$$PV = H(Q) (1 + d + d^2 + \text{----} + d^{Y-1})$$

while X years in the full health state Q^* discounts to PV^*:

$$PV^* = (1 + d + d^2 + \text{----} + d^{X-1})$$

From these two equations we can derive:

$$H(Q) = (1 - d^X)/(1 - d^Y).$$

It is clear that for any H(Q) < 1, X/Y must fall as Y increases.
4 In fact, the *geometric* mean was used; this is somewhat at odds with the principle of giving equal weight to every individual's variations, which would require the *arithmetic* mean to be used.

REFERENCES

Bombardier, C. *et al.* (1982) 'Comparison of three preference measurement methodologies in the evaluation of a functional status index', in R. Deber and G. Thompson (eds), *Choices in Health Care: Decision Making and Evaluation of Effectiveness*, University of Toronto.

Buxton, M. *et al.* (1986) 'Valuation of health states using the time tradeoff approach: report of a pilot study relating to health states one year after treatment of breast cancer', HERG Discussion Paper No. 2, Brunel University.

Christensen-Szalanski, J.J.J. (1984) 'Discount functions and the measurement of patients' values: women's decisions during childbirth', *Medical Decision Making*, 4:47–58.

Farquhar, P.H. (1984) 'Utility assessment methods', *Management Science* 30 (Nov.):1283–300.

Friedman, M. and Savage, L. J. (1948) 'The utility of choices involving risk', *Journal of Political Economy* 56:279–304.

Gudex, C. (1986) 'QALYs and their use by the Health Service', Centre for Health Economics Discussion Paper No. 20, University of York.

Jones-Lee, M., Hammerton, M., and Philips, P. R. (1985) 'The value of safety: results of a national sample survey', *Economic Journal* 95:49–72.

Kahneman, D. and Tversky, A. (1979) 'Prospect theory: an analysis of decision under risk', *Econometrica* 47(2): 263–91.

Llewellyn-Thomas, H. *et al.* (1982) 'The measurement of patients' values in medicine', *Medical Decision Making* 2(4): 449–62.

Llewellyn-Thomas, H. *et al.* (1984) 'Describing health states: methodological issues in obtaining values for health states', *Medical Care* 22(6): 543–52.

Machina, M. J. (1983) 'The economic theory of individual behaviour toward risk', Technical Report No. 433 (Oct.), Institute for Mathematical Studies in the Social Sciences, Stanford University, California.

McNeil, B.J., Weichselbaum, R., and Pauker, S.G. (1981) 'Speech and survival: tradeoffs between quality and quantity of life in laryngeal cancer', *New England Journal of Medicine* 305:982–7.

McNeil, B. J. *et al.* (1982) 'On the elicitation of preferences for alternative therapies', *New England Journal of Medicine* 306:1259–62.

Miyamoto, J. M. and Eraker, S. A. (1985) 'Parameter estimates for a QALY utility model', *Medical Decision Making* 5(1): 191–213.

Pliskin, J.S., Shepard, D.S., and Weinstein, M.C. (1980) 'Utility functions for life years and health status', *Operations Research* 28:206–24.

Raiffa, H. (1968) 'Decision analysis: introductory lectures on choices under uncertainty', Massachusetts: Addison-Wesley.

Rosser, R. M. and Kind, P. (1978) 'A scale of valuations of states of illness: is there a social consensus?', *International Journal of Epidemiology* 7(4): 347–58.

Sackett, D. L. and Torrance, G. W. (1978) 'The utility of different health states as perceived by the general public', *Journal of Chronic Diseases* 31(11): 697–704.

Schoemaker, P. J. H. (1982) 'The expected utility model: its variants, purposes, evidence and limitations', *Journal of Economic Literature* 20:529–63.

Slovic, P. and Lichtenstein, S. (1983) 'Preference reversals: a broader perspective', *American Economic Review* 73(4): 596–605.

Sutherland, H. J. *et al.* (1982) 'Attitudes towards quality of survival: the concept of 'Maximal Endurable Time', *Medical Decision Making* 2(3): 299–309.

Torrance, G. W. *et al.* (1982) 'Application of multiattribute utility theory to measure social preferences for health states', *Operations Research* 30(6): 1043–69.

Torrance, G. W. (1986) 'Measurement of health state utilities for economic appraisal', *Journal of Health Economics* 5(1): 1–30.

Weinstein, M. C. (1986) 'Risky choices in medical decision making: a survey', *Geneva Papers on Risk and Insurance* 11(4): 197–216.

Weinstein, M. C., Pliskin, J. S., and Stason, W. B. (1977) 'Coronary artery bypass surgery: decision and policy analysis', in J. P. Bunker *et al.* (eds), *Costs, Risks and Benefits of Surgery*, Oxford University Press.

Williams, A. (1985) 'Economics of coronary artery bypass grafting', *British Medical Journal* 291:326–9.

Williams, A. (1988) 'Economics and the rational use of medical technology', in F.F.H. Rutten and S.J. Reiser (eds), *The Economics of Medical Technology*, Berlin: Springer.

Part Three

EMPIRICAL PERSPECTIVES

Chapter Seven

ECONOMIC APPROACHES TO MEASURING QUALITY OF LIFE

Conceptual convenience or methodological straitjacket?

ALAN SHIELL, CATHERINE PETTIPHER, NORMA RAYNES, and KEN WRIGHT

INTRODUCTION

There is now widespread acceptance, albeit grudging in some quarters, that the economist has a role to play in the evaluation of welfare services. It is no longer sufficient, if indeed it ever were, simply to consider the effectiveness of programmes; the costs must also be evaluated. This conclusion is not the result of a balance-sheet mentality or preoccupation with pounds and pence but is inevitable given the definition of economic cost. In economic terms the costs of a programme represent the benefits that could have been obtained had the same resources been allocated to another use. An economic appraisal is therefore essentially concerned with comparing the benefits of alternative courses of action. The benefits of social policy are the net effects the intervention is designed to have on the welfare or quality of life of clients. Therefore, to paraphrase one of Harold Wilson's political aphorisms 'one client's quality of life is another client's economic cost'. Far from being the dismal science, economics is concerned with maximizing the benefits we secure from the use of scarce resources. As such there is no contradiction in adopting an economic perspective to quality of life issues.

A further source of disquiet felt by some at the perceived encroachment of the economist into the field of social welfare has more to do with the techniques and methods which are used rather than the alleged preoccupation of the profession. These techniques are founded in neo-classical microeconomic theory and have been developed in more conventional areas such as the analysis of markets and industrial organization. Our purpose in this paper is to consider whether or not techniques such as cost-effectiveness analysis and cost-benefit analysis can be applied sensibly to the evaluation of welfare provision. Can quality of life be measured in a way which facilitates its comparison with hard data such as costs? Is the economist's famed 'bag of tools' an essential item of luggage or just so much excess baggage? These questions are posed in the context of a DHSS-funded study on which the authors have embarked, designed to evaluate the costs and quality of residential services for adults with a mental handicap. We are therefore particularly concerned with the potential advantages and disadvantages of using an economic approach (amongst others) to evaluate the efficiency of services designed to meet the needs of this specific client-group.

The standard economic approach is described in the following section and the importance of measuring outcomes or quality of life emphasized. The shortcomings of the existing measures which have been used to evaluate services for people with learning difficulties are also discussed and consideration is given to the merits of generic quality of life measures which have been used by economists in acute health care settings.

THE PRODUCTION OF WELFARE

Conceptually the economic study of welfare provision draws on an analogy with industrial production. As Figure 7.1 shows, whether it be in the production of industrial goods or residential services, inputs are combined in various ways and in various amounts to produce a quantity of outputs. The outputs are then purchased or otherwise obtained by consumers and used by them to increase their welfare. The term 'inputs' describes the resources required by each production process which, in the case of residential provision, includes both tangible resources, such as the capital and labour required to house and staff each unit, and intangible resources such as the organizational context and level of staff morale. The latter will influence and be influenced by the level of tangible resources but is logically distinct, by definition much harder to quantify and it is questionable whether it can be proxied from conventional sources. The term 'outputs' refers to the results of the production process which, in the example of residential care, is measured initially in terms of the number of resident weeks (or inpatient days) which each unit provides in a specified time period. However, the service provided in each unit is unlikely to be homogeneous and therefore

Figure 7.1   The production of welfare

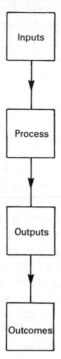

differences in the quality of care must be recognized and incorporated into the model.

This broad framework underpins all economic evaluation but has been refined as the Production of Welfare Model by researchers from the Personal Social Services Research Unit at the University of Kent (Davies and Knapp 1981). Our interpretation of the model differs slightly from that of the Kent team in that we reserve the term 'output' to refer specifically to the immediate results of the production process, i.e. the characteristics of the service. The subsequent effects the use of the service has on the consumer (which the Kent researchers call 'final output') is here referred to as the 'outcome' of welfare provision. This minor semantic difference has the advantage of drawing a clearer distinction between the quality of care (more accurately, the quality of the service) and the client's eventual quality of life. The former relates to the characteristics of each facility and the opportunities which are offered clients, the latter to how the recipient experiences their use, in particular the extent to which the individual feels his or her needs have been met (Raynes 1986). Thus, it is argued here that the two aspects of quality are quite distinct. Others have argued differently, regarding factors such as the environmental features of the unit, the nature of staff-client interaction, and the level of functioning or well-being enjoyed by clients as different perspectives of the residents' quality of life (Hemming *et al.* 1981). Which of these approaches is more correct depends partly on how useful it is to maintain the distinction between outputs and outcomes. For the purposes of this paper the distinction is maintained.

Davies and Knapp (1981) cite three advantages in conceptualizing the production of residential provision in this manner. First, it provides a simple model in which the complex relationships between different inputs and between inputs and outputs can be identified. Second, it provides a technical vocabulary with which these relationships may be discussed. Even if nothing more rigorous than this is attempted, such a conceptual framework offers substantial advantages to practitioners and customers alike. The consumer is returned to the centre of the policy arena because the model requires explicit definition of client-led objectives and much of the sterility which often surrounds policy discussions can be overcome because of the focus on the relative effectiveness and resource consequences of alternative means of meeting objectives. The third advantage, and one from which much of the strength of the model is derived, is the variety of statistical techniques to which the approach lends itself and which can be used to quantify the strength and direction of the relationships between variables.

Thus, for example, it is possible to consider the likely consequences for both cost and quality of adopting different input-mixes, such as nursing or social work qualifications, or different ratios of trained to untrained staff, and to consider the effects of moving from large to small units or vice versa. With a sample of sufficient size multivariate analysis enables the researcher to measure such substitution possibilities and economies of scale with a reasonable degree of confidence and thereby draw conclusions about the relative efficiency of different patterns of service provision. Alternatively cost-effectiveness analysis may be used to assess the relative merits of a small number of alternative policy options relevant to a particular service need.

The analogy between industry and welfare is not complete and the relative importance of measuring the quality of residential provision is partly explained by the differences between the two forms of production process. In industrial production, inputs are purchased and output sold in a series of 'hands-off' transactions at prices determined by the market. It is assumed the firm wishes to maximize profit and therefore its objective is clear and its success easy to measure. The production process whereby inputs are transformed into outputs can largely be ignored and treated as a black box because competitive pressures tend to ensure homogeneous production techniques. The nature of the final outcome may also usually be ignored because for most traded goods and services, outputs and outcomes are made synonymous by the market interactions of fully informed suppliers and consumers. Under the assumption of consumer sovereignty, price, the end result of these transactions, provides a reliable indicator of the value of the goods in question.

The role of the market in the provision of welfare services is less well defined and, where they occur, market interactions tend to be distorted by asymmetries of information or the presence of third parties acting as financial intermediaries. Health care is one area of social policy in which the assumption of consumer sovereignty has been explicitly rejected (Williams 1977). Thus even if market prices were available there is good reason to believe they would not be the most appropriate means of valuing the output of residential provision. The ultimate outcome of services, namely the improvement in the client's quality of life, which the use of the service brings about must therefore be measured and valued directly as an additional exercise.

Neither is it possible to ignore the nature of the productive process. Residential provision is by nature a service and as such it is impossible to separate its production from the act of consumption. Process and output effectively merge into one another. Irrespective of the relative effectiveness of alternative modes of service delivery in terms of the outcome measured at some future point in time, we are not indifferent to what we do to the recipients of welfare services in the process. Perhaps more importantly, it is unlikely that clients are indifferent to the care they receive either. The personal nature of the production process, compounded in this instance by the high likelihood of consumer ignorance about the relative value of the service, means that assessing and monitoring the quality of care is just as important as evaluating its final outcome.

The economic efficiency of a service is described in terms of the relationship between its costs and the final effect its use has on the welfare or quality of life of clients. A cost-effective service is one which either maximizes the improvement in quality of life for a given investment of resources or equivalently minimizes the cost of achieving a given level of welfare. To assess the efficiency of residential provision for adults with a mental handicap it is therefore essential: first to be able to measure quality of life, and second to do so on a comparative basis with costs. Economic costs are defined as the forgone benefits of the next most favoured alternative use of resources but they tend none the less to be measured wherever possible in monetary terms. As a unit of measurement money has certain desirable qualities. In particular, it is measured on a ratio scale and is thus a continuous variable with true zero defining both distance and proportion (Rosser 1983). Ideally the use of the production of welfare approach requires outcome measures which have the same characteristics.

OUTCOME MEASUREMENT IN PRACTICE

The purpose of this section is not to provide a general review of outcome measures but to consider the problem of using existing instruments within an economic framework. Before doing so however, a prior question must be addressed namely: can quality of life be measured meaningfully in a way which allows statistical analysis and explanation in terms of hard data such as costs? A simple answer to this question is no, since one of the drawbacks of a quantitative approach (of which economics is an example) is its failure to incorporate the meaning attached by individuals to the situations in which they find themselves. If quality of life does relate, as defined earlier, to the extent to which an individual feels his or her needs have been met, then this shortcoming may be critical.

Quality of life may be a predominantly subjective concept based on individual values and feelings but it is possible to observe objectively the ascertainable effects of changes in its magnitude. Ideally, it is desirable to assess the effectiveness of services in terms of the clients' perspectives but these are difficult to measure. So little is known about the cost-effectiveness of community residential provision that it does not make sense to ignore the insights provided by a more quantified approach. The weaknesses of the economic approach should be recognized but so also must its strengths. Resource allocation decisions still have to be made, and will continue to be so, irrespective of whether or not information on the efficiency of policy options is available. Value judgements are therefore inevitable and at least by attempting to measure the costs and effects of residential provision the basis for such judgements can be made explicit and subject to debate.

It is possible to identify three ways of measuring the effectiveness of services for people with learning difficulties. Many studies have used measures of the characteristics of residential units as if they were outcome measures on the assumption that the objective of the service is to provide an environment which offers people with a mental handicap the same recognition of their rights and responsibilities as other members of society. It may therefore be considered appropriate to measure the effectiveness of a service in terms of its success in meeting this objective, i.e. the extent to which residential units allow and encourage such recognition. Thus, instruments such as PASS (Wolfensberger and Glenn 1975) and O'Brien's 'Five Accomplishments' (1986) can be regarded as bridging the gap between process and outcome measures. However, they do so only under the plausible assumption that people with a mental handicap share the same values as other members of society and that, irrespective of the degree of disability, culturally valued means remain the best way of meeting their needs.

In other studies proxy indicators have been used to measure something which is believed to be closely related to quality of life. Client engagement (Felce *et al.* 1985) is one widely used example and is regarded here as a proxy measure because it records the external manifestation of an individual's underlying health state rather than his or her own perceptions of how services have been received. While it is plausible that engagement in activities is to be preferred to prolonged inactivity this also remains an assumption which requires testing. With elderly people for example, it has been suggested that some disengagement may be more appropriate (Knapp 1977).

Finally, some researchers have tried to measure directly one or more of the fundamental dimensions of health state. Major domains include physical, psychological, and social well-being and each of

111

these may be broken down still further into sub-categories. Physical well-being, for example, will include self-help skills, mobility, and ability to perform domestic tasks.

Numerous scales exist to measure the cognitive, emotional, behavioural, and physical functioning of people with learning difficulties, the best known of which are the Wessex Behaviour Rating Scale (Kushlick *et al.* 1973) and the Adaptive Behaviour Scale (Nihira *et al.* 1974). The measurement of other psychological and social dimensions of quality of life has progressed further in the context of services for elderly people, where instruments designed to measure life-satisfaction, morale, and self-esteem have been developed (Neugarten *et al.* 1961; Feragne *et al.* 1983). In theory, these instruments could also be applied with some modification to the evaluation of services for people with a mental handicap although there are problems in so doing (Renshaw 1985).

There is, therefore, a wide range of instruments already available which could be used to measure the effectiveness of community residential provision but no instrument is free from problems. To be of any general use the measures must be reliable and valid. Ensuring the validity of instruments designed to measure quality of life is particularly difficult. The results of using different instruments can be compared but ultimately there is no equivalent of the 'gold-standard' to assess whether or not it is quality of life which is being measured. In addition, techniques such as time-sampling are intensive in the use of research time and are therefore expensive to employ. They may also be considered unduly intrusive by staff who are attempting to provide an environment as domestic and home-like as possible – a problem which is often compounded because the most innovative schemes tend also to be the most heavily researched. Finally, there are problems in communicating with some residents which makes the use of interviews with residents and the administration of questionnaires difficult. Obvious problems arise if the resident has a poor concentration span or lacks verbal skills, but less obvious problems also arise. Wyngaarden (1981) has shown that some people with a mental handicap try to please the interviewer by giving what they think is a correct answer or the one which is required by the interviewer. Others tend to acquiesce and answer yes to everything or respond with whatever was the most recently offered option.

These are problems which are general to any attempt to measure the quality of life of people with learning difficulties and will arise irrespective of the professional discipline of the researcher or the methodological framework which he or she chooses to adopt. The difficulties are not insurmountable and may be overcome by, amongst other things, spending time getting to know clients, by using concrete questions, and by using pictures of smiling and unhappy faces to elicit the feelings of people with severe disabilities (Simons 1986). Each of the remedies is time-consuming and requires intensive involvement within each residential facility. Consequently, they would be difficult to fit in to the characteristic Production of Welfare approach which requires a large sample of residential units and, partly because of resource constraints, very little involvement in the operation of each one.

Other problems arise specifically from the attempt to apply an economic framework and use multiple regression techniques to explain differences in the cost-effectiveness of residential units. These include problems in attributing causality as well as difficulties which arise from the use of categorical or individual data and the multidimensional nature of quality of life. Each of these problems is described in greater detail below.

Causality

Conventional economic theory posits that cost is a function of the rate of output which in turn depends on the quantity of inputs and the way they are used. In the analysis of welfare provision the direction of causation is less clear-cut. Quality of care enters as an independent variable, possibly explaining differences in costs, but is in practice often constrained or influenced by, and therefore dependent on, the level of resources previously allocated to the unit. Similar inter-relationships may also be found between staff costs and non-resource inputs such as staff morale. The correlation between the dependent and one or more of the independent variables leads to simultaneous equation bias. Thus, for example, it may be difficult to discern the expected positive relationship between costs and the dependency of residents if staff resources have, in the past, been allocated to units with the most dependent people who are now functioning more capably because of the continued investment of extra members of staff. Cross-sectional data will simply pair off the relatively high staff-resident ratio with the current manifestly low level of dependency and conclude that cost is not a function of the observed capabilities of residents. Time series data is required so that time lags in the relationship between costs, dependency, and changes in outcome may be more appropriately modelled.

Categorical data

Many of the instruments described above, and those used to provide other information of relevance, provide data of a categorical rather than a continuous nature. The National Development Team, for example, classify dependency according to one of four groups ranging from competent in all areas of self help to severe double incontinence, multiple physical handicap, severe epilepsy, etc. It is possible to assign numbers to each group but the classifications are descriptions only and do not define a distance between groups. Thus, an individual in the second group is not twice as dependent as somebody in the first or half as dependent as somebody in the fourth. It is correspondingly difficult to incorporate this sort of information as an explanatory factor in a multiple regression analysis. Either dummy variables must be used, which decreases the explanatory power of the model, or a continuous variable must be constructed, for example by using the proportions of residents who are classified within one or more of the most significant categories.

Individual or group data

With the exception of some environmental quality of care instruments, most outcome measures provide individual scores for each resident. Cost information, on the other hand, tends to be unit or facility based. As many of the resources of a residential unit are shared between the residents it is very difficult to apportion the costs to individuals in any way which is meaningful and not arbitrary. An alternative means of reconciling cost and outcome data is to aggregate the individual scores and calculate an average for the unit as a whole. However, there are also obvious problems with this practice. For categorical data it will be impossible to calculate a unit average other than implicitly; based on the researcher's subjective impression of the unit taken as a total entity, with all the problems of reliability that such a gestalt-process implies. For some variables, such as gender, it is simply meaningless to calculate an average of any sort.

Even for continuous variables, the use of average scores is not without problems, for it ignores the information provided by the variance. Age is one example, where any effect on the cost of provision is more likely to arise from the proportions of residents who are either very old or very young rather than the average age of all residents which would usually be employed in multiple regression analysis. The degree of variation in care practices within a residential unit may also be quite large and can lead to problems even with instruments which are already unit based. The Group Home Management Schedule (Pratt *et al.* 1980), for example, classifies units according to the extent to which they are resident- or institution-oriented. Many large facilities are now subdivided into small semi-autonomous sub-units and, whether because of differences in the capabilities of the residents or in the attitudes of the staff, care practices may vary substantially from one group to another. In some facilities integral ex-staff accommodation is used to provide some residents with a large degree of independence and autonomy extending even to total control over personal finances. Yet others, within the main body of the unit, possibly but not necessarily because of the extent of their disabilities, are unable to exercise such control. This variability makes it difficult to rate a residential unit according to the extent to which residents as a whole are involved in decision-making processes and domestic activities.

Multi-dimensional outcomes

Neither quality of life nor quality of care are unidimensional concepts and therefore many researchers employ a battery of instruments to provide a profile of the individual or institution. This obviously provides more information than the use of a single indicator but can lead to problems if reductions in one dimension are associated with improvements in another. Unless there is some means of assessing the relative value of each dimension, thereby allowing trade-offs to be made, it becomes impossible to evaluate the overall effectiveness of the service in question or compare its efficiency with alternative means of meeting the same needs.

A UNIVERSAL MEASURE OF HEALTH OUTCOME

The general paucity of outcome measures is one reason why economic techniques have not had more widespread use in the health field and therefore it is not surprising that economists have been involved in the development of measures more suited to their needs. This involvement has centred around the quality adjusted life year (QALY) which is a universal measure of health status (Kind *et al.* 1982).

Conceptually the QALY offers a number of advantages over other measures of outcome although the existing instrumentation has been criticised (see Loomes and McKenzie in this volume). These criticisms point to the need for continued research and development, but our concerns are more specifically related to the problems of applying the concept to the evaluation of services for people with mental handicaps. The first of our concerns is whether policy objectives relate to health improvements or to the acquisition of skills which are more common to education than health policy. This is not to deny the importance of the improvement and maintenance of the health of people with a mental handicap, but rather to regard their health care in the same way as the rest of the population and to regard the care and training which occurs in residential services as a means of improving personal development. The essential point of such a change in emphasis is to relate improved functioning to personal development potential. If this were done, a move from one level of functioning to another would not necessarily be of the same value for each individual.

The second issue is one which is common to many long-term care sectors and involves once again the question of whether environmental qualities are part of or distinct from final outcome. It could be argued that the provision of a comfortable, safe, domestic environment is an important objective of policies which provide residential facilities for people unable to make their own arrangements, in which case the QALY measure does not have a set of categories to measure its achievement.

Finally, there is the question of whose health state is important as the provision of services will have an effect not only on the immediate users but also their family, friends, and neighbours. Theoretically, there is no problem considering such 'externalities', but the logistical problems of doing so are enormous.

CONCLUSION

The Production of Welfare approach offers two main advantages to those with an interest in the planning, management, and evaluation of services for people with learning difficulties. First, as a simple model of the relationship between available resources and the provision of services designed to meet the pre-specified needs of clients, it provides a useful framework for policy discussions, facilitating co-operation between the various agencies and, by restoring the client to the centre of the policy arena, helping to break down barriers caused by professional self-interest. Second, as an analytical tool, it can quantify the relationship between inputs and outputs and lend empirical weight to any proposals which emerge from the subsequent negotiations.

To exploit these advantages to the full it is essential to measure the quality of life of people with mental handicaps, ideally in a way that allows comparisons to be made with the costs of services designed to meet their needs. This is certainly a difficult task but is not one which is impossible.

We have argued that the Production of Welfare approach does offer useful insights and may indicate ways in which services can be delivered more effectively and efficiently. But this does not mean that it is the only way of evaluating service provision nor that it is necessarily the best. The insights it offers are essentially quantitative and, though substantive, are restricted by the type of data the model must use. The importance of some non-resource inputs, such as the organizational context in which care is delivered, the actual processes whereby resources are transformed into outputs, and the residents' own perceptions of the value of the services they receive may each be under-represented or even omitted from the analysis. The Production of Welfare approach complements other methods and does not subsume them at all. It must be supported wherever possible with information of a more qualitative nature. This will raise further methodological problems about how best to incorporate the information from the two sources of enquiry but these are unlikely to be insurmountable though they indicate the need for a multidisciplinary approach. The end result of such co-operation will be a greater understanding of what is involved in improving the quality of life of people with mental handicaps and more efficient use of the resources needed in the process.

REFERENCES

Davies, B. and Knapp, M. (1981) *Old People's Homes and the Production of Welfare*, London: Routledge & Kegan Paul.

Felce, D., DeKock, U., Saxby, H., and Thomas, M. (1985) *Small Homes for Severely and Profoundly Mentally Handicapped Adults Final Report*. Southampton Health Care Evaluation Research Team, University of Southampton.

Feragne, M. A., Longabaugh, R., and Stevenson, J. F. (1983) 'The psychosocial functioning inventory,' *Evaluation and the Health Profession* 6(1): 25–48.

Hemming, H., Lavender, T., and Pill, R. (1981) 'Quality of life of mentally retarded adults transferred from large institutions to new small units,' *American Journal of Mental Deficiency* 86(2): 157–69.

Kind, P., Rosser, R., and Williams, A. (1982) 'Valuation of the quality of life: some psychometric evidence', in M.W. Jones-Lee (ed.) *The Value of Life and Safety*, Amsterdam: Elsevier/North Holland.

Knapp, M. (1977) 'The activity theory of ageing: an examination of the English context', *Gerontologist* 17:553–9.

Kushlick, A., Blunden, R., and Cox, G. (1973) 'A method for rating behaviour characteristics for use in large scale surveys of mental handicap', *Psychological Medicine* 31:466–75.

Neugarten, B. L., Havighurst, R. J., and Robin, S. S. (1961) 'The measurement of life satisfaction', *Journal of Gerontology* 16:134–43.

Nihira, K., Foster, R., Shellhaas, M., and Leyland, H. (1974) *Adaptive Behaviour Scale*, 1974 Revisions, Washington.

O'Brien, J. (1986) *A Guide to Personal Futures Planning*, Atlanta Georgia: Responsive Systems Associates.

Pratt, M. W., Luszcz, M. A., and Brown, M. E. (1980) 'Measuring dimensions of the quality of care in small community residences', *American Journal of Mental Deficiency* 85:188–94.

Raynes, N. (1986) 'Approaches to the measurement of care', in J. Beswick, T. Zadic, and D. Felce (eds) *Evaluating the Quality of Care*, BIMH Conference Series.

Renshaw, J. (1985) 'Measuring outcomes for mentally handicapped people', PSSRU Discussion Paper 304/2, University of Kent.

Rosser, R. (1983) 'Issues of measurement in the design of health indicators: a review', in A. Culyer *Health Indicators*, London: Martin Robertson.

Simons, K. (1986) 'Kirklees Relocation Project Environmental Evaluation Schedule', University of Sheffield.

Williams, A. (1977) 'Measuring the quality of life of the elderly', in L. Wing, and A. Evans (eds) *Public Economics and the Quality of Life*, Johns Hopkins University Press.

Wolfensberger, W. and Glenn, L. (1975) *PASS – Program Analysis of Service Systems: Handbook, Field Manual*, 3rd Edn, Toronto National Institute of Mental Retardation.

Wyngaarden, M. (1981) 'Interviewing mentally retarded persons: issues and strategies', in R. H. Bruininks, C. E. Meyers, B. B. Sigford, and K. C. Lakin (eds) *Deinstitutionalization and Community Adjustment of Mentally Retarded People*, AAMD monograph 4: Washington D.C.

Chapter Eight

SPOUSE CARERS
Whose quality of life?

GILLIAN PARKER

INTRODUCTION

The arguments in favour of care for people with disabilities and chronic illnesses taking place within, and being provided by, the community are by now so well rehearsed that they have almost become part of the 'given' world. Notwithstanding the occasional question-mark raised by feminist commentators (Dalley 1983; Finch 1984) or the occasional hiccup created by the speed or practicalities of decarceration (Jones and Poletti 1986) there appears to be a broadly based consensus that care in the community is good, care at home is better, and care by the family is best.

Indeed, the evidence tends to support this assumption. When working well, care at home and by the family *is* best for people who are ill or disabled: for example, elderly people cared for at home live longer (Davies and Challis 1986), people with multiple sclerosis adapt better and show more gains in rehabilitation when supported by their families (Power 1985), polio sufferers return home sooner when they have a ready-made support system (Creese and Fielden 1977), and so on. We all 'know' these things, but we also 'know' – but usually keep the knowledge in a separate compartment – that these benefits to the disabled or ill person are bought at a cost which neither often nor in any large part falls to the state. The cost of care in and by the community is borne largely by the family and usually by its female members (see Parker 1985). Thus gains in quality of life for one member of a family or household almost inevitably mean reductions in the quality of life of others. In order to answer the question, 'Whose quality of life?', then, one has to be able to dis-aggregate costs and benefits within the family and household unit.

120

The nature of caring for children with disabilities and its impact on parents has been described and examined in some detail in the past ten years (e.g. Baldwin 1977, 1985; Wilkin 1979; Glendinning 1983, 1985). Similarly, the burdens borne by those caring for frail elderly people, particularly those who are mentally disturbed, have now been documented by several researchers (e.g. Gilleard and Watt 1982; Nissel and Bonnerjea 1982; Levin *et al.* 1983; Wenger 1984; Jones and Vetter 1985) and there is more research in progress. However, the position of those who care for non-elderly disabled adults, particularly when the carers are spouses, has not received the same amount of attention from researchers, or, indeed, policy makers.

The disaggregation of costs and benefits within marriage or marriage-like relationships appears to pose problems for researchers, policy makers, and service providers alike. This difficulty arises only in part from the general 'carer-blindness' that has existed until very recently because, as indicated above, this 'blindness' is proving capable of remedy. Rather the difficulty arises largely from implicit assumptions held about the unitary nature of marriage and marital relationships. Husband and wife are assessed as a single unit for tax and social security purposes; the concept of the 'family wage' still exists and still depresses women's remuneration in the labour market; research on poverty and resources concentrates on 'tax units' or households and assumes that all members share resources equally; two are assumed to be able to live as cheaply as one – especially when the two are married; and so on. Further, movement away from the idea of the family or household as a 'black box', within which emotional, practical, and financial transactions remain hidden and unresearchable, has been slow.

Although research informed by feminism has started to challenge these assumptions (see, for example, Brannen and Wilson 1987) there is a long way to go before the different needs and expectations of both partners in marital relationships are automatically considered separately by researchers or policy makers. Yet such considerations are absolutely vital in respect of couples where one member is disabled. While the costs of caring are most difficult to disentangle in the case of spouse carers, when ideological barriers to the very idea of such disentanglement are overcome and methodological problems solved, it is here that the differential costs of disablement and caring are likely to be thrown into most relief.

121

THE IMPACT OF DISABLEMENT IN MARRIAGE

Evidence for a causal relationship between measures of stress and the role of informal carer is fairly conclusive but evidence about the particular aspects of the caring task which contribute most to raised stress levels is equivocal (see Parker 1990). However, several studies do show that the role of *spouse* carer is particularly stressful. For example, carers of people who have suffered head injuries experience very high levels of stress immediately after the initial injury and continue to display higher than normal levels one and two years later (Oddy *et al.* 1978; Livingston *et al.* 1985b). This stress level is closely related to the current functioning of the injured person. For spouse carers, however, stress both starts, and remains, at a higher level than for other carers and they experience a higher degree of 'psycho-social handicap' (Livingston *et al.* 1985a). In the case of cardiac arrest spouses are actually more distressed than are patients during hospital admission (Mayou *et al.* 1978). Further, the sooner patients return to work – a measure of positive outcome from the point of view of health professionals – the greater the stress experienced by their spouses, with higher reported levels of depression, anxiety, and tiredness. Similarly, spouse carers of those who have suffered a stoke have a higher incidence of minor psychiatric disturbance than do other types of carers and this is particularly evident when the stroke has resulted in aphasia (Kinsella and Duffy 1979).

The relationship between aphasia and distress in spouse carers gives a broad hint about one of the *causes* of this stress. Evidence from studies about head injury, aphasia, and Huntington's chorea shows that it is the loss of a relationship between 'equals' that makes caring for a spouse so problematic. Changes in personality associated with these conditions cause the greatest strain as the previously 'equal' partner becomes a 'pseudo-child' (Korer and Fitzsimmons 1985). If the carer can effect his or her own transformation into a 'pseudo-parent' then it becomes easier to cope. If this transformation is not possible – and for spouses it usually is not – then stress results. Not surprisingly, then, the mothers of head-injured patients find it easier to accept the changes in behaviour and personality which reduce their (typically) sons to an earlier stage of dependence (Thomsen 1974; Rosenbaum and Najenson 1976; Oddy *et al.* 1978; Livingston *et al.* 1985a). Further, parents' reactions can also increase the difficulties which spouses experience:

> These tensions [with patient's parents] were often aroused by the
> in-laws' overprotective attitude toward their son ... many of the
> brain-injured men exhibited childlike dependency behavior.
> Parents may have found such ... behavior quite gratifying while
> they were slipping back to the old parent-child relationship. For
> the wife, on the other hand, who had never known her husband
> as a child, such behavior was quite aversive.
>
> (Rosenbaum and Najenson 1976:887)

Thus parents 'regain' a child while a spouse 'loses' a husband or
wife – but the spouse has no opportunity to mourn this loss:
'Although [s]he has lost [her]his mate as surely and permanently as
if by death, since the familiar body remains society neither recognizes the spouse's grief nor provides the support and comfort that
surrounds those bereaved by death' (Lezak 1978:593). Relationships
between carer and the cared-for person are put under strain even
when the impact on personality is not as devastating as in head-
injury, stroke, or Huntington's chorea.

Spouse carers carry a larger burden than any other type of carer
(except, perhaps, the single carer of a dependent elderly person or
mentally handicapped adult – but this is a shrinking group) simply
because they have no one else with whom they can share it. While
the parents of children with disabilities may not share the caring
tasks equally (Cooke 1982; Glendinning 1983) at least they can
divide between them the responsibilities of breadwinner and housekeeper. The spouse carer has no such choice unless he/she is able to
earn enough to pay someone else to take on housekeeping responsibilities. Wives of men who become disabled or ill in mid-life find
themselves taking on a whole range of responsibilities of which they
have had no previous experience and for which they may be physically ill-equipped (Finlayson 1973; Rosenbaum and Najenson 1976;
Mayou et al. 1978; Korer and Fitzsimmons 1985). The same is
undoubtedly true of the husbands of women who become disabled.

Similarly, spouse carers have no one with whom to share the
financial burden of caring. Cartwright et al. (1973) showed that in
the 12 months before the death of the cared-for person, husbands
and wives who were principal carers were more likely than any other

group of carer to experience changes in their employment pattern. Very few employed spouses reported *no* changes in their paid work but wives were more likely to have been affected than husbands. In addition, wives were more likely to have given up paid work altogether to care for their husbands whereas husbands caring for their wives tended to cope by taking time off work.

This pattern is not surprising: in two-partner households caring for a disabled relative 'rational' decisions about which partner, if either, should give up or forgo paid employment, based on economic considerations, can be made. When one partner in a couple becomes ill or disabled no such element of choice exists. When the main breadwinner (usually the husband) is affected it is difficult, if not impossible, for the other partner to replace his earnings. If it is the main housekeeper (usually the wife) who is affected then the breadwinner may be forced to give up his job or reduce his hours of work in order to care for her, their children, or both.

Despite this some spouse carers do attempt to fulfil both roles at considerable cost to themselves. Sainsbury (1970) reports that younger non-disabled wives usually felt impelled to take on full-time employment to support their household even if they were only marginally better off as a result.

At the same time as income falls expenditure increases to meet the needs of the disabled person (Hyman 1977). Given that these extra needs are to some extent immutable or unnegotiable it is inevitable that the carer spouse will carry the additional burden of reduced spending on *his* or *her* needs.

Although both partners will usually be aware of the financial constraints produced by disablement, their perceptions of the role of money may be very different. Thompson and Haran (1984) give a graphic example of this in their study of amputees and their carers: 'amputees who declared their income to be inadequate were usually wanting financial recompense for the loss of the leg, whereas helpers needed the money to pay the bills!' (Thompson and Haran 1984:289).

This difference in perspective spread to other aspects of the couples' lives. The amputees sought social activity largely to escape from the confines of their homes: for their carers 'it represented an opportunity to salvage some kind of normality for their nuclear family unit' (Thompson and Haran 1984:289).

This effect on 'a broader spectrum of relationships and roles' is particularly evident in regard to spouse carers' social and family lives. When a partner suffers a stroke, and particularly when it is accompanied by aphasia, spouses experience a decrease in contact with *their* friends, impaired leisure activities and generally diminished social interaction (Kinsella and Duffy 1979). Friendships frequently falter altogether. Thompson and Haran (1984) similarly found a high level of social isolation among carers of amputees which grew greater over time. Carers had a great need for social activity but no one enabled them to fulfil this need. This social isolation was particularly important not just because it was a substantial cost for the spouse carers to carry but also because it seemed to suppress the carers' ability to express any need.

This reduction in the spouse's social life is not due solely to the difficult practicalities of going out. Even when the disabled spouse can be safely left at home or alternative care arrangements made, the carer spouse has substantial attitudinal barriers to surmount:

> The spouse lives in a social limbo, for [s]he does not have a
> partner with whom [s]he can participate in social activities, nor is
> [s]he free to get one. Today's social milieus tend to consist
> mostly of couples or singles: the single spouse fits into neither.

> (Lezak 1978:593)

For most, the effort required to overcome these barriers proves too much:

> You feel very much apart ... and after the years you don't really
> belong anywhere. You just don't join in anything really. It's a
> funny barrier that comes in. You're on a different wavelength
> because although you've got a husband you haven't.

> (Murray 1985:22)

The loss of shared social activities, the practical burden of care, the emotional stress, the financial impact of disablement, and the lost or changed relationship between the partners puts inevitable strain on the marriage. Sexual relationships can deteriorate or stop altogether (Rosenbaum and Najenson 1976; Lezak 1978; Kinsella and Duffy 1979) and not always solely as a result of the physical constraints imposed by disablement. All the other elements of change,

125

particularly those which alter the balance between 'equals', also contribute. It becomes increasingly difficult for the spouse who has to provide a great deal of intimate physical care to a partner to continue seeing him or her as a sexual partner:

> It is not easy for the disabled [partner] to be both patient and sexual partner in a relationship which now involves both, or for [his or] her [spouse] to fulfil the role of nurse and lover. The emotional switch is very subtle. The nurse (as an example of a 'carer') employs touch in a very special way and for specific purposes, and she is permitted very intimate contact only by maintaining emotional distance from the patient.... When one's spouse takes on nursing functions, a curious relationship shift takes place as the role becomes polarised into 'nurse' and 'patient'. When this polarisation is fixed, sexual relationships are sure to founder. Both partners are caught in a double bind from which it is difficult to escape without psychological assistance.

(Campling cited in Stewart 1985:277)

The inevitable outcome of all these demands on the marriage and the partners is, for some at least, separation and divorce.

The evidence on the incidence of divorce after the adult onset of disability is equivocal but this seems to have much to do with the different samples and research techniques used in different studies. What does seem to emerge is that if marriages are going to break up they do so fairly rapidly after the onset of disability (Sainsbury 1970; Blaxter 1976; Silver *et al.* 1985).

Another pattern which emerges from studies is the particular susceptibility of younger married couples to break-up of their marriage (Sainsbury 1970; Silver *et al.* 1985). Explanations for this effect have included the possibility that some degree of disablement is expected the older one becomes therefore, for older married couples, the adjustment required is not so great (Sainsbury 1970). However, it seems possible that this pattern may emerge as a result of the *nature* of disablement prevalent in different age groups. Younger people are more likely to suffer a traumatic and sudden onset, through head – or spinal cord – injury, therefore their marriages may fail quickly. Older people suffer more from slowly degenerative conditions and therefore have more time to adjust to the changes brought about. Older couples may, therefore, not break up as spectacularly as do younger couples but may, after many years, be left with a relationship that is a marriage in name only.

CONCLUSION

The aim of this chapter, like that by Baldwin and Gerard (Chapter Nine, this volume) has been to show that the impact of disablement or ill-healthy is not confined solely to the person who suffers from it. The case of carers who are married to the person they care for illustrates this vividly yet, until very recently, has received little attention. The evidence presented here shows again that the costs borne by carers are certainly qualitatively, and probably also quantitatively, different from those borne by the people they care for.

New research at the Social Policy Research Unit has added significantly to this evidence. In this project 21 non-elderly couples have been interviewed in depth about the impact that the disability or chronic illness of one of the partners has had on their lives in general, and on their marriage in particular. The partners have been interviewed separately as well as together and the analysis concentrates on their different experiences and the different costs that they bear (Parker 1992). I have not attempted to suggest here any ways of redressing the costs which spouse carers bear. Rather, I have tried to raise in readers' minds some doubts about the advisability of measuring the quality of life of any single individual without also taking into account the quality of life of those who support and care for him or her.

If these doubts are reasonable then they leave us with a series of methodological problems, applicable in all fields – not just in relation to spouses – the most important of which seem to be:

(a) how do we develop measures which give us *comparable* information on costs for the carer and the cared-for person? For example, is the cost of the loss of paid work for the person with the disability equivalent to the cost of the loss of paid work for the carer?

(b) how do we assign weights to the cost of disablement *vis-à-vis* the cost of care. For example, are the benefits to the carer of taking paid work outside the home – the release from caring tasks, the opportunity to meet people outside the household, the financial independence it might bring – to be assigned less or more importance than the costs which the carer's going out to work imposes on the person with the disability?

(c) how do we build in to assessments of the quality of life a longitudinal element which goes beyond life expectancy to take into account the fact that increases in the quality of life for the disabled or sick person *now* may be bought at the risk of the eventual break-down of the caring situation, i.e. when the costs to the carer have caused her or him to give up caring?

REFERENCES

Baldwin, S. M. (1977) *Disabled Children – Counting the Costs*, London: Disability Alliance, Pamphlet no. 8.

Baldwin, S. M. (1985) *The Costs of Caring*, London: Routledge & Kegan Paul.

Blaxter, M. (1976) *The Meaning of Disability*, London: Heinemann.

Brannen, J. and Wilson, G. (eds) (1987) *Give and Take in Families: Studies in Resource Distribution*, London: Allen & Unwin.

Cartwright, A., Hockey, L., and Anderson, J. L. (1973) *Life before Death*, London: Routledge & Kegan Paul.

Cooke, K. (1982) *1970 Birth Cohort – 10 year follow-up study: Interim Report*, University of York, Department of Social Policy and Social Work: Social Policy Research Unit Working Paper DHSS 108/6.82 KC.

Creese, A. L. and Fielden, R. (1977) 'Hospital or home care for the severely disabled: a cost comparison', *British Journal of Preventive and Social Medicine* 31:116–21.

Dalley, G. (1983) 'Ideologies of care: a feminist contribution to the debate', *Critical Social Policy* 8:72–82.

Davies, B. and Challis, D. (1986) *Matching Resources to Needs in Community Care*, Aldershot: Gower.

Finch, J. (1984) 'Community care: developing non-sexist altenatives', *Critical Social Policy* 3(3):6–18.

Finlayson, A. (1973) *Role Rearrangement by Married Women after Familial Crises*, SSRC Grant Report, HR 846/2.

Gilleard, C. and Watt, G. (1982) 'The impact of psychogeriatric day-care on the primary supporter of the elderly mentally infirm', in R. Taylor and A. Gilmore (eds) *Current Trends in Gerontology: Proceedings of the 1980 Conference of the British Society of Gerontology*, Aldershot: Gower.

Glendinning, C. (1983) *Unshared Care*, London: Routledge & Kegan Paul.

Glendinning, C. (1985) *A Single Door*, London: George Allen & Unwin.

Hyman, M. (1977) *The Extra Costs of Disabled Living*, Disability Income Group/Action Research for the Disabled Child.

Jones, K. and Poletti, A. (1986), 'The "Italian experience" reconsidered', *British Journal of Psychiatry* 148:144–50.

Jones, D. A. and Vetter, N. (1985) 'Formal and informal support received by carers of elderly dependents', *British Medical Journal* 7/9/85:643–5.

Kinsella, G. J. and Duffy, J. D. (1979) 'Psychosocial readjustment in the spouses of aphasic patients', *Scandinavian Journal of Rehabilitation Medicine* 11:129–32.

Korer, J. and Fitzsimmons, J. S. (1985) 'The effect of Huntington's Chorea on family life', *British Journal of Social Work* 15:581–97.

Levin, E., Sinclair, I., and Gorbach, P. (1983) *The Supporters of Confused Elderly People at Home: Extract from the Main Report*, London: National Institute for Social Work Research Unit.

Lezak, M. D. (1978) 'Living with the characterologically altered brain injured patient', *Journal of Clinical Psychiatry* 39:592–8.

Livingston, M. G., Brooks, D. N., and Bond, M. R. (1985a) 'Three months after severe head injury: psychiatric and social impact on relatives', *Journal of Neurology, Neurosurgery, and Psychiatry* 48:870–5.

Livingston, M. G., Brooks, D. N., and Bond, M. R. (1985b) 'Patient outcome in the year following severe head injury and relatives' psychiatric and social functioning', *Journal of Neurology, Neurosurgery, and Psychiatry* 48:876–81.

Mayou, R., Williamson, B., and Foster, A. (1978) 'Outcome two months after myocardial infarction', *Journal of Psychosomatic Research* 22:439–45.

Murray, N. (1985) 'I used to long to go away by myself for a few days', *Community Care* 1/8/85.

Nissel, M. and Bonnerjea, L. (1982) *Family Care of the Handicapped Elderly: Who Pays?* London: Policy Studies Institute.

Oddy, M., Humphrey, M., and Uttley, D. (1978) 'Stresses upon the relatives of head injured patients', *British Journal of Psychiatry* 133: 507–13.

Parker, G. (1990) *With Due Care and Attention: A Review of Research on Informal Care*, London: Family Policy Studies Centre Occasional Paper no. 2 (second edition).

Parker, G. (1992) *With This Body: Caring and Disability in Marriage*, Buckingham: Open University Press.

Power, P. D. (1985) 'Family coping behaviors in chronic illness: a rehabilitation perspective', *Rehabilitation Literature* 46 (3–4):78–83.

Rosenbaum, M. and Najenson, T. (1976) 'Changes in life patterns and symptoms of low mood as reported by wives of severely brain-injured soldiers', *Journal of Consulting and Clinical Psychology* 44 (6):881–8.

Sainsbury, S. (1970) *Registered as Disabled*, Occasional Papers on social administration no. 35, London: Bell & Sons.

Silver, J. R., Oliver, M. J., and Salisbury, V. (1985) *The Long-Term Effects of Spinal Cord Injury: An Interim Report* (mimeo).

Stewart, W. (1985) *Counselling in Rehabilitation*, London: Croom Helm.

Thompson, D. M. and Haran, D. (1984) 'Living with an amputation: what it means for patients and their helpers', *International Journal of Rehabilitation Research* 7(3):283–92.

Thomsen, I. V. (1974) 'The patient with severe head injury and his family: a follow-up study of 50 patients', *Scandinavian Journal of Rehabilitation Medicine* 6:180–3.

Wenger, C. (1984) *The Supportive Network: Coping with Old Age*, London: George Allen & Unwin.

Wilkin, D. (1979) *Caring for the Mentally Handicapped Child*, London: Croom Helm.

Chapter Nine

CARING AT HOME FOR CHILDREN WITH MENTAL HANDICAPS

SALLY BALDWIN and KAREN GERARD

INTRODUCTION

Thalidomide created a watershed in public awareness of disability in childhood and the impact it can have on family life. When the Thalidomide affair erupted in the early 1970s it quickly became clear that reliable information on the numbers of children with disabilities, their situation and that of their families was completely lacking. Even very severe disability in a child was a virtually invisible phenomenon, though advances in medical techniques were enabling children who would previously have died to survive into adulthood. When acknowledged at all by professionals and policy makers, childhood disablement was regarded as unproblematic, subsumed into the private domain of the family or assumed to be adequately dealt with by social and medical services. Thalidomide destroyed that complacency, bringing to light the profound difficulties experienced by the great majority of children with disabilities and their families and the inadequacy of the support they received (Bradshaw 1980).

Public awareness has been heightened further by the growing impact of 'community care' as a government theme for organizing formal support for people with disabilities over the last two decades. The theme stresses the desirability of maintaining people with disabilities in their own homes or, where this is not possible, enabling them to live in accommodation and occupy homes as similar as possible to those available to the rest of the population (see, for example, DHSS 1971, 1980). In a sense community care policy is less relevant to children with disabilities, the great majority of whom have always been looked after by their families. However, a significant number of mentally handicapped children have, in the past, lived in long-stay hospitals. There is now a clear government commitment to ensuring that mentally handicapped children do not spend their lives in long-stay hospitals. In future, then, such children will be cared for 'in the community' – the majority living with their families as they have always done. That this is now actively promoted by government as the preferred mode of care to some extent makes the informal care supplied by families more visible; creating, in theory at least, a clearer obligation to assess how the long-term care of a child who is disabled affects the family's quality of life and to provide appropriate support.

EFFECTS ON FAMILIES

Our knowledge of childhood disability and its effects on family life has increased considerably since the Thalidomide episode. We are now able to document more systematically how disablement in a child affects families and to think more clearly about appropriate policy interventions. The research undertaken over the last 15 years has demonstrated that the long-term care of a disabled child can profoundly affect the quality of life of the whole family and also that it can affect different family members in very different ways. The experiences of mothers, for example, have been shown to differ greatly from those of fathers and siblings (Hewett 1970; Kew 1975; Wilkin 1979) while the disabled child's own experience may be quite different from that of other family members. Nor need the experience be simple or uniform. Families vary in their response. The care of a child who is disabled frequently creates heavy burdens, however many families report that their disabled child brings particular kinds of happiness and satisfaction for the family. Hence in discussing how disability in a child affects a family's quality of life it is important to distinguish between effects on particular individuals and on the family unit as a whole and to distinguish positive and negative effects. As we note below, the methodological problems of doing this are considerable.

This chapter is concerned with children who are mentally handicapped, concentrating on the costs, in the widest sense of that term, created by their day-to-day care and on ways of mitigating these. This is not to deny that, like all children, those with mental handicaps bring pleasures and rewards. Rather the assumption is that for such pleasures to survive it is probably necessary to remove as many of the burdens of care as possible. To do this means knowing what they are. The chapter reviews the evidence on the effects of disablement on various aspects of the family's and the child's quality of life. We go on to consider the role of policy interventions whose objective is to reduce family stress and the necessity of evaluating these in the light of their benefits and costs for the disabled child, as well as for other members of the family. In so doing we draw on findings from research undertaken in the Social Policy Research Unit and in the Centre for Health Economics at the University of York.

What *are* the costs of caring for a child who is mentally handicapped? The research evidence suggests that these can usefully be grouped under four headings: physical, opportunity, financial, and psychological costs.

Physical costs

Severe disability creates dependency far beyond the normal dependencies of childhood. Until they are three or four, most children need help with washing, dressing, eating, and other aspects of self-care. Many will not be fully continent; most will need occasional attention in the night. However, as a large body of research now demonstrates, severe mental handicap in a child intensifies and prolongs these dependencies. As Table 9.1 shows, children with mental handicaps can remain highly dependent.

Hirst's work on young adults with disabilities shows that similar levels of dependency persists well into adult life. Of Hirst's sample of

Table 9.1   Dependency in self-care – children with mental handicaps, aged 5–15

Help:	A moderate amount needed %	A great deal needed %
Washing	11	81
Dressing	15	82
Feeding	39	49
Toileting	50	32
Attention at night	20	62
Supervision by day	34	58

Source: Baldwin (1985): data re-analysed by Baldwin, Godfrey, and Haycox.[1]

133

young mentally handicapped people aged 16 to 22, 66 per cent were unable, for example, to stay safely at home alone for an hour, while 89 per cent were unable to travel alone on a public bus (Hirst 1983).

Caring for children with this degree of dependency is very taxing physically. Coping for long periods with what Bayley (1973) terms 'the daily grind' of care, not only lifting, toileting, and feeding, but also the increased laundry and other house work created by incontinence, sickness, and behaviour disturbance, is hard and debilitating work particularly when sleep is regularly disturbed. Many parents report effects on their own health such as backache and high blood pressure, while the necessity of providing such continuous high levels of care and supervision inevitably restricts the lives of parents and other children in a large number of ways.

Opportunity costs

One set of restrictions concerns opportunities for social and leisure time, both for parents themselves and for the family as a whole. For the principal carer – almost invariably the child's mother – the child's need for care and supervision inevitably means the loss of opportunities for leisure time – for doing things they would otherwise do such as reading, watching television, going out socially, even sleeping. Interviews with mothers (see Glendinning 1983) demonstrated the frustration of being unable, for example, to attend evening classes, study for A levels or train for a new career. There are also costs for other family members, since behavioural problems can create difficulties in taking family holidays and going on outings. Parents have less free time to spend on other children, while the mentally handicapped child's needs or behaviour can create difficulties in inviting friends home, or in finding time or space to play quietly. There are also, as already noted, benefits. Some of the mothers in Glendinning's study identified particular pleasures and satisfactions they gained in being able to meet the disabled child's special needs and thought their other children gained a great deal from the experience. To acknowledge these benefits is *not*, however, to say that they somehow cancel out the costs.

For mothers one of the more significant opportunity costs is the curtailment of opportunities for employment outside the home. In Baldwin's (1985) research, for example, women with a mentally handicapped child were much less likely to be in paid employment than the women in a control group drawn from the general population (30 per cent as against 59 per cent), or, when they were, to work as many hours (20 as against 24 hours a week). This was true for mothers of children of all ages. As children grew up and the women in the control group went back to work, the differences became much more pronounced. Effects on fathers' employment were less clear. Men with a mentally handicapped child were not, for example, less likely to be in paid work, though the career prospects of men in professional occupations did appear to have suffered.

The economic significance of these findings is discussed below. What is stressed here is their psychological significance. It is widely recognized that employment outside the home has important meanings quite apart from its function of generating income. It provides opportunities to meet people socially, to act in different roles from those played at home, to structure one's time, to make achievements. For women these functions of paid work can be even more important than for men. Ungerson (1981) for example, argues that while men view the home as a refuge from the pressures of paid work, women see in paid work an opportunity to escape from the repetitive and isolating routines of housework and child care. For a woman with a severely mentally handicapped child the value of paid employment in providing an escape from home will be of even greater importance. Detailed, qualitative work with women caring for disabled children indicates that this is indeed so (Wilkin 1979; Glendinning 1983). On the other hand little or no information is available on the extent to which the morale of fathers is affected when their employment suffers. Baldwin's (1985) research suggested that the effects were slight; those men who would have minded effects on their career tended to prevent this from happening.

Financial Costs

Earnings

Effects on employment opportunities are likely to affect earnings. Baldwin's research, which used the Family Expenditure Survey (FES) to compare the incomes and expenditure patterns of families with and without a disabled child, found clear evidence of such effects. The earnings of women with a mentally handicapped child in this study who were in paid employment were, on average, £6.60 a week less than those of similar women in the control group; those of non-manual male workers were on average £12.10 a week less. The joint weekly earnings of families with a mentally handicapped child were £17.70 a week less, on average, than those of control group families though this narrowed to a difference of £4.10 a week in their disposable incomes when benefits paid on account of the child's condition had been taken into account (all at 1978 figures). These differences relate to all families with a severely mentally handicapped child. They were considerably higher among families with older children. At this point in the family life cycle mothers in the control group were increasingly in full-time employment and fathers reaching their earnings peak. Among the families with a mentally handicapped child, by contrast, life-cycle earnings profiles were essentially flat, remaining at levels characteristic of families with very young children.

Extra costs

The figures presented above take no account of any extra costs generated by disablement. However a mass of evidence now demonstrates clearly that mental handicap *does* create such costs: for example, transport for children unable to use public transport; clothing and bedding destroyed by incontinence, dribbling, or aggressive behaviour; wasted food and toys that are destroyed; special equipment or house adaptations (see, for example, Buckle 1984). It is simple to identify categories of expense in this way. The methodological problems of measuring them precisely are, however, enormous: the choice of time periods to which expenditure should relate; the choice of method, given the weaknesses of both subjective accounts and observation of expenditure; the interpretation of data—dealing with items that cannot be afforded, for example, or are only met via economies by other household members. To cope with some of these problems Baldwin's study used a mix of behavioural and subjective methods. Over 85 per cent of the families with a mentally handicapped child in her study reported that they had extra costs because of the child's condition: regular everyday costs; less frequent and larger 'capital' costs, and 'crisis' costs arising from hospital admissions (Baldwin 1985).

There were clear differences between the everyday expenditure of the families with a mentally handicapped child and those of the control group. The former spent more of their total income each week, the extra going on items like food, children's clothing, transport, and household equipment. The level of extra expenditure varied with incomes, hence it is not possible to talk of an *average* cost borne by families with a mentally handicapped child. Families in the middle income range spent an average of £5.80 a week extra in 1978 (around £15 at 1988 prices) while families in the lowest income range spent an average of £6.40 a week extra, and those in the highest range an average of £15.05 (around £16 and £38 at 1988 prices).

To these costs must be added larger, more intermittent, costs such as house adaptations and specially purchased consumer durables. For Baldwin's sample as a whole, an average of £184 had been spent on such items during the preceding two years (roughly £500 at 1988 prices). Many families had also incurred substantial costs in connection with hospital admissions. It was not thought sensible to average such costs, however where they did occur, families' finances were disrupted for a considerable period of time – not only by paying for transport to hospital and buying things for the child but by loss of earnings, child minding for other children, and lack of time to budget as they would normally have done.

The overall effect

Given the variation that exists in families' capacities for extra expenditure, in their preferences, and in the characteristics of their children's disabilities, the wisdom of combining figures on earnings loss and extra costs to produce a global estimate of the overall financial impact of mental handicap is dubious. It should be borne in mind, however, that extra costs have to be met from incomes that are constrained by caring for the child. Inevitably then, families' living standards are lower than they might otherwise have been. Parents in Baldwin's study described what this meant for them: fewer luxuries than their peers enjoyed – no holidays abroad or in hotels but always in caravans or self-catering accommodation; fewer new clothes for parents; waiting longer to replace a car; no new fitted kitchens or furniture renewed when children were older; fewer evenings in the pub; bills never paid till the final demand; little or no savings. Some parents found it difficult to talk about deprivations they or their other children experienced because this looked too much like complaining or, worse, blaming the disabled child.

Others were forthright that they *were* poorer because of their child's condition and that money *was* important. It could help to make a difficult life easier. Finding money, for example, for a mother to have driving lessons and a small car of her own, could utterly transform *her* life and benefit the rest of the family accordingly.

Psychological costs

The evidence that caring for a child who is severely mentally handicapped causes emotional and psychological strain is abundant, whether it takes the form of subjective accounts by parents or psychological/psychosomatic indicators. Parents identify two broad 'causes' of stress: background anxieties or difficulties, and specific incidents which trigger episodes of anxiety or depression. For example, they are frequently emotionally ground down by dealing with the child's behaviour and have continuous anxieties about what will happen to him or her when they die or are unable to cope. Stress may also be caused because of worries about the way the disabled child's condition affects their other children; difficulties in getting out or having any time for themselves; frustration at their inability to return to paid work; or constant worries about money. In addition to these chronic background problems parents also identify particular stress points: a birthday which highlights their child's failure to reach a 'normal' developmental milestone; a bout of illness or admission to hospital; difficulties in obtaining services or benefits; unsympathetic treatment by people in shops or restaurants (Glendinning 1983).

The measurement of stress is notoriously difficult. A significant body of research, nevertheless, has been concerned with measuring and exploring variations in the stress levels of parents with a severely disabled child (see, for example, Chetwynd 1985; Quine and Pahl 1985). This work shows clearly that the stress levels of mothers with a mentally handicapped child are significantly higher than among women in the general population. (Again, virtually no work has been done on fathers' stress levels.)

However, variations in stress levels are considerable and difficult to explain. Work by Bradshaw and Lawton (1978) and Hirst (1985), for example, found no strong association between mothers' stress levels, the nature or severity of the child's disability, and a range of socio-economic factors. Parker (1985) on the other hand, re-

138

analysing Bradshaw and Lawton's (1978) data, identifies factors which do appear to exacerbate or ameliorate mothers' stress levels. This analysis suggests a number of practical policy interventions through which the psychological stress arising from the care of a child who is mentally handicapped might be relieved. Many of these interventions point to the need for relief, in one way or another, from the continuous responsibility for supervision and care.

REDUCING THE COSTS?

Given the kinds of cost identified above, and their likely impact on the quality of life of carer, cared-for, and other family members – and given an acceptance that such costs should not be borne wholly by the families concerned – the logical question to address is what can be done to reduce their impact and enhance the quality of life of all or some of these 'clients'? In terms of social and fiscal policy, a wide range of responses is possible at both the individual and macro levels: from the tailoring of highly specific packages of support to more general measures such as income maintenance and housing policies. However, relatively little appears to be known about the appropriateness of particular interventions or their effectiveness in alleviating the burdens of care.

As noted above, one need commonly expressed by parents is for a break in the continuous routines of care and supervision. Respite care services provide one form of response to this need. In the remainder of this chapter we draw on the available research evidence to assess how effective this particular form of statutory response to the needs of families with a mentally handicapped child appears to be.

EVALUATING RESPITE CARE

Respite care may be provided in one of three settings: residential, short-term fostering schemes, or domiciliary care. Residential care requires the person cared for to be taken into care by the providing agency. Short-term fostering, on the other hand, centres around the provision of substitute families to do the caring, whilst domiciliary care supports the carer in their own home.

Whatever the mode of delivery, the general aims are similar: to provide a break for the carer from the unrelenting 'daily grind' of care and supervision.Guidelines produced by the National Children's Bureau (Robinson 1984) clearly state the objectives of respite care: optimally it should not only produce a break for the carer from the physical and emotional strains of long-term dependency but should improve the quality of life of all family members including the mentally handicapped child. A minimal requirement should be to ensure that the mentally handicapped child is at least no worse off by receiving this care, whilst the carer at least benefits from the breaks.

Clearly it is important to evaluate the different forms of respite care, not only from the point of view of understanding situations in which one form of respite care is more appropriate than another but also more generally, since respite care is one element in a potentially wide range of interventions available to be combined together to provide individually tailored community care 'packages'.

Evaluation of respite care should be considered therefore in terms of its success in achieving its stated objectives. However the evidence reviewed below reveals that very little is known about the proven worth of such care, despite a growing receptiveness on the part of formal care providers to invest in the development of respite care policies. An underlying cause of this present state of knowledge comes from problems arising early in the evaluation process. Enumerating and measuring the impact of respite care on all parties affected remains a complex task, still in embryonic form.

The most commonly described and measured effect of respite care on carers' quality of life is the relief of carers' stress (e.g. Butler *et al.* 1982; Quine and Pahl 1985). The measurement of stress is probably the most sophisticated development that evaluation studies in this area have used, although an understanding of the underlying relationship between stress and caring is, as already noted, incomplete (Parker 1985). Regarding other areas of quality of life, it has been only relatively recently recognized that the impact on the mentally handicapped child's life should be considered (Oswin 1984). In this area too, quality of life measures are at an early stage of development (Kind 1988).

Furthermore the evidence already obtained reveals an imbalance in the amount of research according to the mode of respite care. There are, for example, a considerable number of studies on the effectiveness of residential-based respite care but much less on which to draw for the effectiveness of short-term fostering schemes or domiciliary services.

Residential respite care

Residential services usually take the form of either 'specialist' (i.e. short stay only) or 'mixed' (i.e. catering for both short stay and long term) provision. Conflicting evidence has been produced by surveys on the effectiveness of residential respite care. Younghusband *et al.* (1970) found that relief from the care of the mentally handicapped child at home was the most pressing of personal and social needs. In an evaluation of short-term hostel care Vaughan (1979) found that such resources were proving a valuable help for families to keep their children at home. However, Oswin's study (1984) was critical of this service which has developed over the past 30 years with no national plan but from responses to innovation and the enthusiasm of local parents and professionals. She recognized it as an important specialist resource but one which should be used carefully. As a result of observational analysis Oswin was critical about the quality of life for the mentally handicapped child whilst in such care. Her criticisms include the mixing of children using residential services for short-stay and long-term care, on the grounds that it is extremely difficult for staff to meet the needs of both groups adequately. Furthermore, she disputed that very young children (i.e. under five years old) should be separated from their families. Indeed too much respite care, she believed, was built upon the untested premiss that separation of the child and family is 'good'.

As part of Pahl and Quine's work on effectiveness of respite services (Pahl and Quine 1984), parents in two neighbouring health districts were interviewed. Satisfaction was high (94 per cent and 81 per cent respectively for the two districts) although many of the parents were reluctant to ask for respite care initially because of the sense of failure or shame they felt about their child being taken into care. Parents were particularly concerned about the quality of the care and stimulation given to their child during their stay. They saw the benefits of this care as mainly for their children rather than for themselves.

In a study by Gerard (1988) parents using respite services were asked to represent both their own views about the service and its value for their mentally handicapped child. Table 9.2 below summarizes these responses in terms of the difference respite care made to family life and to the individual well-being of the mentally handicapped child.

The impact on the quality of life of the family was perceived to be

Table 9.2   Impact of respite care on quality of life

Difference in quality of life	Family % of respondents (n = 146)	Mentally handicapped child % of respondents (n = 146)
Better	78	78
Worse	1	5
Indifferent	17	15
No response	4	2

high by the majority of users (78 per cent thought respite care improved the situation). However a minority of respondents (17 per cent) claimed that respite care made no difference to family life. As advocates, parents were generally in agreement that their mentally handicapped child also benefited from the service (78 per cent thought that they did). This was achieved through the scope for wider social contact which was thought both to stimulate recreational activities and promote both physical and emotional independence. For those remaining parents who did not think their child benefited (22 per cent), 15 per cent found it impossible to articulate either way on the matter. Only five per cent of respondents felt the service directly affected their child adversely. These data may therefore indicate a conflict of interests for a sizeable minority of users of respite care.

Parker (1985) summarizes the current state of the literature on residential respite services, viewing it as mainly responding to carers needs but poorly evaluated in terms of direct effects on carers or dependents. On a more positive note she claims that this picture is slowly beginning to change as awareness about community care generally grows.

Short-term foster care

Short-term foster care provides surrogate parents for the mentally handicapped child to stay with in a 'home from home' environment. Evidence available on short-term foster care has attracted variable reaction from researchers. Since these schemes start from the premiss that it is better for a child to be kept within a family environment than in residential care, such schemes accord with the general principles of community care. The pioneering schemes set up in Leeds and Somerset have proved very successful (Freeman 1977;

Toyne 1978). Robinson's research (1986) provides a detailed account of one short-term foster scheme in Avon. This evaluation portrays a generally positive response in terms of the benefits which accrue to the children (e.g. socialization) but at the same time qualifies this with evidence that some children have negative reactions (e.g. home-sickness). Such schemes therefore require constant monitoring to select out children with negative responses and consider alternative forms of support for them and their families. Thus, although the Avon study showed that there was a sizeable group of children who remained homesick or demonstrated other negative responses (e.g. refusing to eat), the majority (two-thirds) of parents felt their children were able to broaden their horizons and social circles by doing new things and meeting other people when staying with the foster family.

The effect of the Avon scheme on family life in the child's paren-tal home was described in terms of 'a sense of relief' (66 per cent), 'more time and attention for other children' (10 per cent), and 'having more time for each other' (18 per cent). Others thought the scheme had a preventive effect by 'keeping parents sane', and by helping parents to continue caring for the child at home (7 per cent). In contrast only 3 per cent of the families felt the scheme made little or no difference to their lives.

Domiciliary care

The third type of setting for respite care is within the child's own home. A hybrid, unskilled, community worker (i.e. a cross between a home help, nurse, and sitter) visits the family home and offers help with whatever the carer specifies. The approach is designed to be flexible and responsive to individual family needs. There is very little evidence from published sources concerning the nature of the impact on carers' or their dependants' lives, although some general monitoring and assessment has taken place (e.g. Cooper 1985).

In summary, attempts at evaluating respite care highlight some of the general problems encountered in the evaluation of services aiming to support both carer and cared-for within one family simultaneously. At the theoretical level it may be possible to separ-ate the correlates of stress arising directly from the caring role from those of other stress-producing activities in a carer's life. If so it would be possible to assess the direct impact of respite care. (There is an alternative view that the relationship between stress and a carer's quality of life is multifactorial, hence individual causal relationships cannot be identified.) However, even if it were possible to assess the impact of respite care on the carer's welfare it seems unlikely that its direct impact on the welfare of the child could also be assessed. To do this is theoretically possible but would require very large samples, whereas in practice (and by definition) community care is fragmented, making identification of large groups of like people extremely difficult. Moreover respite care is usually one of several services received by the mentally handicapped child. Other services include specialist education and, in some cases, specialist socal work services. These services will contribute simultaneously to the child's development, making it difficult to disentangle the separate effects of individual services and the direction of causality in relationships between service receipt and quality of life. This will be even more challenging in the case of respite care as its pattern of use will be intermittent, making its effect open to interaction with and contamination by the other services received.

On the most extreme scenario therefore, neither carer nor caredfor can be rigorously assessed in terms of the direct impact respite care has on their own quality of life. How then *can* it be assessed? Perhaps its role should be seen in palliative terms, in which case any contribution respite care makes to reduction in stress among parents or to improvements in independence and socialization on the part of the child should be counted as the benefits of the service.

Problems also remain in operationalizing the trade-off in the welfare of the client groups involved, and in finding out what service would be the most suitable for a child who is mentally handicapped. It remains unclear how the very difficult dimensions of benefits and disbenefits accruing to mentally handicapped children and their families should best be traded against each other, especially when their interests may conflict. It is suggested by Oswin that such a conflict is likely to be significant in determining carers' and childrens' quality of life.And how, in practice, can the views of the children be elicited? Obtaining the relevant information from people who are mentally handicapped can be problematic in itself; this is compounded by the fact that the service users in this case are children. Parents are the usual choice of advocate for children. However, using them in this case raises the potential problem that their own views may conflict with, and more importantly override, their children's. Ideally other advocates should be used, while observation techniques can also provide useful information. There may also be value in adapting behaviour scales to understand the impact of respite care on the child's welfare. This has not been attempted in current approaches, but could be one focus of emerging research on measuring quality of life in children.

Further development of research techniques is therefore required to measure the benefits of respite care services. To pick up the important changes possibly effected by respite care, measures are needed which are not only reliable and valid, but also highly sensitive. Important but intangible benefits/disbenefits include the impact of mixing short-term respite care within a long-stay home on both groups of children; the effects of respite care on other family members, notably siblings; and the effects of short-term fostering on the foster family. To develop these components of the methodology presents great challenges, however the work of Robinson (1986) indicates that they are not insurmountable.

CONCLUSION

This chapter has shown that the costs experienced by families caring for mentally handicapped children are significant and diverse, potentially affecting the quality of life of all members of the family. Community care policy assumes that such children will optimally live with their families, however it is generally accepted that the costs and diswelfares arising from their care should not fall completely on the families concerned; a collective responsibility exists to provide support which eases the burden of care. In practice this responsibility can be exercised via social and fiscal policies operating at either the macro or the individual level: through income maintenance mechanisms for example, or through social work support and services in kind.

It would always be desirable to assess the appropriateness and effectiveness of interventions which aim to relieve stress and improve the quality of life of mentally handicapped children and their families. Current resource constraints make this an increasingly urgent task. However much more is known at present abut the costs of care than effective ways of alleviating these.

This chapter has demonstrated that one aspect of policy, respite care, has an important role to play in reducing some of the stress associated with the care of children who are mentally handicapped.

At a very general level, respite care appears to be considered useful by parents of mentally handicapped children. However on-site evaluation has not to date provided a clear account of its impact on all parties concerned. This chapter has argued that in order fully to evaluate the effects of respite care it is necessary to face up to the difficult task of trading off gains and losses in the quality of life of different family members. While this is not an insurmountable task the process of identifying and measuring the impact of respite care on all the people involved is, as noted in the chapter, still at an early stage. Assessing its impact on the mentally handicapped child's quality of life, for example, remains at a descriptive stage while the impact on siblings and spouse-partner relationships are only now beginning to be described.

Respite care is, moreover, only one of a number of possible policy interventions. Families respond to mental handicap in a child in their own individual way, developing particular caring routines and coping strategies. The needs of some may be met more appropriately by financial support or adequate housing or by enabling mothers to go out to work, rather than by the provision of respite care as such.

It is necessary, then, for policy makers to recognize the individual nature of families' needs for support and, by extension, their individual perception of the costs and benefits of different types of intervention. This suggests a policy based on an individual approach to the assessment of need. The right to an assessment of individual needs is a central feature both of the Griffiths Report on Community Care (Griffiths 1988) and of the new Disabled Persons (Services, Consultation, and Representation) Act 1986, currently in the first stages of implementation. Recognizing this right will clearly require the formal sector to accept its own role in ensuring that the costs of disability are not left to lie completely where they fall.

NOTE

1 Baldwin's (1985) study included children with a wide range of disabling conditions. This chapter draws on an unpublished analysis of the study data relating to children with handicaps, undertaken by Baldwin, Godfrey, and Haycox. This analysis also utilized data from research by Haycox and Wright to compare the costs of caring for children with mental handicaps in a range of public and private settings.

REFERENCES

Baldwin, S. (1985) *The Costs of Caring*, London: Routledge & Kegan Paul.

Bayley, M. (1973) *Mental Handicap and Community Care*, London: Routledge & Kegan Paul.

Bradshaw, J. (1980) *The Family Fund: An Initiative in Social Policy*, London: Routledge & Kegan Paul.

Bradshaw, J. and Lawton, D. (1978) 'Tracing the causes of stress in families with handicapped children', *British Journal of Social Work* 8(2): 181–92.

Buckle, J. (1984) *Mental Handicap Costs More*, London: Disablement Income Group.

Butler, N. R., Haskim, M., Stewart-Brown, S., *et al.* (1982) *Child Health and Education Study: First Report on the 10 year follow up*, Department of Child Health: University of Bristol.

Chetwynd, M. (1985) 'Factors contributing to stress in mothers caring for an intellectually handicapped child', *British Journal of Social Work* 15:295–304.

Cooper, M. (1985) *Hard-won Reality: An Evaluation of the Essex Crossroads Care Attendant Schemes*, Essex County Council Social Services Department.

DHSS (1971) *Better Services for the Mentally Handicapped*, Cmnd 4683, London: HMSO.

DHSS (1980) *Mental Handicap: Progress, Problems and Priorities*, London: HMSO.

Freeman, J. (1977) *Mental Health and Community Care: A Scheme Devised in Leeds*, Social Work Service Report no. 14.

Gerard, K. (1988) 'Costs and effects of respite care for families with mentally handicapped children', paper presented at Health Economists' Study Group, University of Newcastle upon Tyne, 6–8 January.

Glendinning, C. (1983) *Unshared Care*, London: Routledge & Kegan Paul.

Griffiths, Sir R. (1988) *Community Care: Agenda for Action*, London: HMSO.

Hewett, S. (1970) *The Family and the Handicapped Child*, London: Allen & Unwin.

Hirst, M. A. (1983) 'Evaluating the malaise inventory: an item analysis', *Social Psychiatry* 18:181–4.

Hirst, M. A. (1985) 'Young adults with disabilities: health employment and financial costs for family carers', *Child: Care, Health and Development* 11:291–307.

Hirst, M. A. and Bradshaw, J. (1983) 'Evaluating the malaise inventory: a comparison of measures of stress', *Journal of Psychosomatic Research* 27:193–9.

Kew, S. (1975) *Handicap and Family Crisis*, London: Pitman.

Kind, P. (1988) 'The design and construction of quality of life measures', Discussion Paper no. 43, Centre for Health Economics, Health Economics Consortium, University of York.

Oswin, M. (1984) *They Keep Going Away: A Critical Study of Short-Term Residential Care Services for Children who are Mentally Handicapped*, King Edward's Hospital Fund for London (Report).

Pahl, J. and Quine, L. (1984) *Families with Mentally Handicapped Children: A*

Study of Stress and of Service Response, Health Services Research Unit, Uniersity of Kent at Canterbury.

Parker, G. (1985) 'With due care and attention: a review of research on informal care', Occasional Paper no. 2, London: Family Policy Studies Centre.

Quine, L. and Pahl, J. (1985) 'Examining the causes of stress in families with severely mentally handicapped children', *British Journal of Social Work* 15:501–17.

Robinson, A. (1984) *Respite Care Services for Families with a Handicapped Child*, London: National Children's Bureau Briefing Paper.

Robinson, C. (1986) *Avon Short Term Respite Care Scheme: Evaluation Study – Final Report*, University of Bristol, Department of Mental Health.

Toyne, R. (1978) *Partnership with Parents: Short Term Care for Handicapped Children in Somerset*, Taunton Social Services Department.

Ungerson, C. (1981) *Women, Work and the 'Caring Capacity of the Community': Report of a Research Review*, Social Science Research Council.

Vaughan, P. J. (1979) 'An evaluation of short-term hostel care', *Apex* 7(3): 76–7.

Wilkin, D. (1979) *Caring for the Mentally Handicapped Child*, London: Croom Helm.

Younghusband, E., Birchall, D., Davie, R., and Kellmer Pringle, M. L. (eds) (1978) *Living with Handicap*, London: National Children's Bureau.

Chapter Ten

SECURITY AND AUTONOMY
*Criteria for judging the quality of care offered to
adolescents in time-limited placements*

CELIA DOWNES

In this paper, I argue that quality of life is dependent on the quality
of relationships available to a person and which they have the capacity to sustain. For many adolescents in foster care, it is the capacity to make relationships which has been stunted. A prerequisite
for enlarging this capacity is that foster parents make themselves
reliably available at a critical period in the adolescent's development. In order to develop criteria for judging the quality of care
offered by foster parents, it is necessary to focus on aspects of the
relationship which develops between them and the adolescent placed
with them.

Adolescence is a time for exploring the world outside the family.
By this means, a realistic appraisal of one's own capacities and those
of other people develops. Adolescents who have developed thus far
with secure attachments may take it for granted that this exploration
is part of the process of separating from their family of origin and
becoming self-reliant young adults. This is largely because they are
able to experience their family as a secure base for exploration, to
which they may return from time to time when they feel the need.
They will also be developing other, new attachments which in time
will take over the function of the secure base from the family of
origin.

Autonomy in adolescents and adults is not being understood to
mean absolute self-reliance, without recourse to other people. The
position taken in this paper follows that of Attachment Theory,
which draws attention to the phenomenon that:

> human beings of all ages are happiest and able to deploy their
> talents to best advantage when they are confident that, standing

behind them, there are one or more trusted persons who will come to their aid should difficulties arise. The person trusted, also known as an attachment figure (Bowlby 1969), can be considered as providing his or her companion with a secure base from which to operate.

(Bowlby 1979)

A number of studies notably into the etiology of adult mental disorders, (Brown and Harris 1978; Henderson 1982; Parkes 1982) and into marital separation (Weiss 1982) support this view. For a person to have the experience of a secure base from which to operate, there needs to be a trustworthy figure or figures available and willing to help if called upon. Additionally the person concerned needs to be able to recognize the trustworthy figure as such and as available and willing to help, and must also be able to collaborate so that an effective alliance is formed.

The powerful influences of repeated past experiences of educational and social failure and of unreliable attachment figures leave many adolescents in care overwhelmed by age-appropriate psychosocial tasks. In the course of the research on which this paper is based (Downes 1986, 1988), three such tasks were identified as particularly preoccupying adolescents in time-limited foster care. These were, first, negotiating the transition to outside school or work as a step on the way to establishing themselves as adult workers; second, discovering, exploring, and coming to terms with feelings about their birth families and other previous significant carers and testing out their likely future reliability; third, negotiating around the end of the placement in relation to leaving home.

Achieving autonomy, as defined above, was the preferred outcome in the research on which this paper is based. It has been argued that for this to develop, the adolescent in care first needs to be offered a reliable relationship. He or she also needs to enter into an alliance with one or both foster parents if the relationship is to be experienced as a secure base for exploration. Through the research it was possible to identify some criteria for judging the quality of the relationship that foster parents offer. In order to do this, it focused on foster parents' statements about the purposes and significance of the placement, their agenda in relation to the adolescents' preoccupations, outlined above, their evaluation of the success or failure of the placement. The consistency of the foster parents' agenda and the degree to which it was openly, explicitly shared with the adolescent or remained hidden, was also examined.

It was found that placements where foster parents openly shared their purposes and evaluations with the adolescent were those where there was considerable overlap between the foster parents' and adolescent's agenda, particularly with respect to the adolescent's wish for continuity with previous relationships. In these placements the foster parents' agenda was coherent and consistent and there was agreement with the adolescent on their evaluation of the success of the placement. These placements ran for their planned length and were experienced as mutually satisfying, with the parties remaining in contact after the placement ended. In contrast, in placements where there was little shared meaning and a large measure of hidden agenda, the foster parents' agenda was often directly opposed to that of the adolescent, particularly with respect to the adolescent's wish for continuity with previous relationships. The foster parents regarded the placements as failing. The placements ended earlier than had been planned, they were experienced as mutually unsatisfying and none remained in contact with each other.

FOSTER FAMILY PLACEMENT FOR ADOLESCENTS IN CARE AS A ROUTE TO INDEPENDENT LIVING

Specialist fostering projects providing time-limited placements for difficult adolescents in care have constituted a significant development in social work practice since the mid-1970s. The adolescents concerned would previously have been considered 'unfosterable' by social workers. Those who entered care in adolescence usually found their way via Assessment Centres to Community Homes with Education; less frequently they were to be found in Secure Units or in Adolescent Units attached to psychiatric hospitals. Those considered difficult, who had been in care for a number of years, were likely to have experienced a series of moves between smaller community homes, residential special schools, and foster care.

It was in the course of acting as a consultant to one such project that I became intrigued by the interactional processes associated with success and those associated with failure. Like similar projects elsewhere, the project generated a sense of optimism among participating social workers and foster parents. Yet at the same time it was clear that this was a risky, emotionally demanding venture for all concerned. Social workers found they could not predict the course or character of a placement. Some adolescents, whose behaviour had previously proved very difficult for residential social workers, settled down and were no trouble, while with others, difficult behaviour came to light for the first time in family placement. Those taking part could not fail to question the wisdom of placing within a family previously unknown to them, adolescents who either had little experience of family life, or highly unsatisfactory experiences of parental care. Would it not be wiser to put resources into developing independent living units while providing training in 'survival skills', rather than expecting adolescents to attach themselves to a new family at an age when their contemporaries were preoccupied with separating from their family of origin?

A BRIEF SUMMARY OF THE RESEARCH METHODOLOGY

The project on which the research was based provided placements intended to last between 6 months to 2 years for adolescents in care aged between 14–17 years on entry who were assessed as 'difficult' enough. The sample consisted of 23 placements. One sub-sample of 11 was studied prospectively at 3-month intervals through their placements, providing a means of noting changes over time. Another sub-sample of 12 was studied retrospectively at the point the placement ended.

Data were collected through family group interviews. This allowed for two kinds of data analysis. First, it was possible to get accounts of what had been happening in the family from what persons said. Second, it was possible to develop an understanding of family interactions by observing behaviour, participation patterns, sequences, and the like. Family group interviews were used for all interviews with the prospective sample. This was not always possible with the retrospective sample, for example, if a placement broke down abruptly. Therefore parallel forms of a semi-structured inter-view schedule were devised that could be used with adolescent and foster family together or separately.

Interviews were an hour long and were recorded on audio tape. They were open ended and relied on a few key questions. In this kind of interview the inteviewer cannot be a bystander who is unin-fluenced by events or ignored by the family. This was acknow-ledged: both the ways in which the family sought the interviewer's involvement, and the impact of events in the course of the interview, became part of the data which required attention and analysis. When the analysis of the interviews was complete, a brief search of the adolescents' case records was made. Its purpose was to complement the anecdotal accounts with a brief chronological history and family tree. The interviews were completed between 1979 and 1983.

A sequence of data analysis steps was devised and applied consistently across the data. These moved step by step between the raw data and eventual conceptualization. To start with, full transcripts were prepared, then the data were extracted and combined in a variety of ways to make visible their contents. Charts and diagrams were used to depict data.

The findings related to the meanings attributed to the placements by the foster parents are summarized in Tables 10.1 and 10.2. Table 10.1 shows foster parents' agenda and evaluation of placements. Table 10.2 shows foster parents' evaluative perceptions of adolescents through placements.

DISCUSSION OF FINDINGS

Agenda set by foster parents concerning psycho-social tasks in the placement identified as important to the adolescents

In all the placements, foster parents saw it as part of their job to help the adolescent back into school, or into work (see Table 10.1, col. 3). In thirteen placements an agenda was formulated which supported the adolescents' sense of continuity with the past, and their wish to reappraise their relationships with members of their own family and other previous carers and to test out whether there would be a home-base for them when they left care. By contrast, foster parents' agenda in nine placements implied that the purpose of the placement was to discourage continuity with the past. It will be seen from Table 10.1, cols 4 and 5 that there were agenda in three placements pointing in each direction. These indicated a change of agenda over time as events unfolded.

In thirteen placements an agenda was formulated in terms of building up and maintaining a relationship which would keep the door open for the adolescent to maintain contact with foster parents once the placement was over, and the adolescent no longer in care. This included encouraging the adolescent to live near the foster

Table 10.1 Foster parents' agenda and evaluation of placements

		Agenda					Evaluation			
1	2	3	4	5	6	7	8	9	10	11
Foster parents	Adolescent	Agenda relating to help with school or work	Agenda to support the adolescent's sense of continuity with the past	Agenda encouraging discontinuity with the past	Agenda encouraging continuity with foster family	Agenda to end placement earlier than first planned	Placement evaluated a success	Placement evaluated a failure	Placement evaluated as too short for maximum benefit	Aspects of policy and practice of project blamed
Armstrong	Tim Larkin	*			*		*		*	
	Mark Robinson	*	*		*				*	
	Wayne Brett	*	*					*		
	Andy West	*	*		*		*		*	
	Tom Skipper	*	*		*		*		*	
	Paul Elliott (ii)	*	*			*		*		
Campbell	Wendy Bell	*			*		*			*
Goldman	Kevin Flynn	*	*					*		*
Hatton	Dawn Gibson	*				*				
	Christine Faber	*	*		*			*		
	Mandy Shepperd	*	*	*	*			*	*	
	Julie Piggett	*		*	*			*	*	*
Harding	Paul Elliott (i)	*		*				*		
Henderson	Clare Dobson	*	*			*		*		*
	Gina Fitzgerald	*				*		*		
	Diane White	*	*	*			*			*
Knight	Veronica Williams	*	*	*	*			*	*	*
Murphy	Rose Phillips	*	*		*			*	*	
	Frank Little	*	*			*		*	*	*
Page	Eddie Lewis	*		*	*	*		*	*	*
Rushmoor	Vicky Jones	*	*		*		*		*	
Wilkinson	Lee Robinson	*		*	*			*		
	Ben Little	*		*					*	

Table 10.2   Foster parents' evaluative perceptions of adolescent through placement

Name of foster parents	1 Foster parents progressively perceive adolescent as a destructive person	2 Foster parents perceive adolescent as a mixture of a destructive person, a victim of circumstances, and as unmotivated for the placement	3 Foster parents perceive adolescent as making progress during the placement, but also a victim of circumstances, and destructive	4 Foster parents perceive adolescent as making progress during the placement
Armstrong	Wayne Brett	Mark Robinson Paul Elliott (ii)		Tim Larkin Andy West Tom Skipper
Campbell				Wendy Bell
Goldman	Kevin Flynn			
Hatton		Dawn Gibson Julie Piggett Paul Elliott (i)	Mandy Shepperd	Christine Faber
Harding				
Henderson	Clare Dobson Gina Fitzgerald			
Knight			Diane White Veronica Williams	
Murphy		Frank Little	Rose Phillips	
Page		Eddie Lewis		
Rushmoor			Vicky Jones	
Wilkinson		Lee Robinson Ben Little		
	4 placements	9 placements	5 placements	5 placements

home. In six placements, an agenda was formulated which indicated that the foster parents aimed to end the placement earlier than
first planned (see Table 10.1, cols 6 and 7).

*Foster parents' evaluation of the placement as a whole, and of the adolescent
placed with them*

One of the most striking findings was that in only six placements did
the foster parents evaluate the placement a success. While in thirteen placements their evaluation was in terms of failure. In the
others no verdict was offered (see Table 10.1, cols 8 and 9).

Four general themes were identified from the evaluative
comments made by the foster parents about the adolescent placed
with them:

1. Perceptions of the adolescent's destructiveness or sabotaging
behaviour. Such behaviour was seen as either aimed at the foster
parents and their children, or at other fostered adolescents, or at
the success of the placement.
2. The adolescent as victim of past circumstances and/or
current relationships.
3. The adolescent as unmotivated for foster family placement.
4. The adolescent as making progress during the placement.

Placements could be grouped according to which theme pre-
dominated, or whether the foster parents' perceptions were more
mixed. These groupings are shown in Table 10.2.

By combining these data with those in Table 10.1 some interesting
comparisons begin to emerge, particularly between groups 1 and 4
of Table 10.2. In group 1 all four placements are evaluated as
failures. There is no agenda to remain in contact with the adolescent
once the placement ends, and no evaluations that the adolescent
would have benefited from a longer placement. All instances of an
agenda to end the placement earlier than originally planned fall
within groups 1 and 2. In contrast, in group 4, four out of five placements were evaluated a success, and in all cases the agenda was to
keep in touch once the placement ended. In groups 3 and 4 all but
one offered agenda items concerned with supporting the adolescent's sense of continuity with own family and past carers.

Clearly, foster parents' perceptions of adolescents making 'progress', however defined, colour their wish and intentions to keep in contact with them, and their evaluation of the placement. The way a foster parent defines progress in an adolescent will be influenced by the agenda they have set in the first place.

From the foster parents' attributions of meaning to the placement, we turn to consider some of the implications of the meanings expressed and the way they were expressed. A summary of the researcher's evaluations are given in Table 10.3.

The consistency or inconsistency of the foster parents' agenda

I would expect this to be important, in determining the outcome of the placement, given the general aim of providing a secure base for exploration for adolescents who hitherto have had poor experience of the reliability of attachment figures. Note that agenda evaluated as coherent or consistent is not necessarily also evaluated as appropriate or helpful.

In fourteen placements the foster parents' agenda appeared coherent and consistent, and in nine placements to lack coherence and consistency to a marked degree. In three families where more than one adolescent was studied, consistency (Armstrongs and Murphys) or inconsistency (Hendersons) appeared to be a pattern. Two others (Wilkinsons and Hattons) presented as consistent in some placements: inconsistent in others (see Table 10.3, cols 3 and 4).

The most common pattern of inconsistency, found in six placements, was for the initial agenda to be set at an unrealistically high or unconditional level in terms of the total commitment of the foster family. Having failed to spell out conditions and consequences of behaviour at the start, there was the almost inevitable change of agenda when the adolescents' behaviour took foster parents to the limits of their tolerance. For example, Diane White, who had been 'taken as their daughter' by the Hendersons, was threatened with being cut off totally if she decided to go and live with her drug-addicted boyfriend. In two other placements the inconsistency was between the foster parents' stated agenda for influencing the adolescent's behaviour and what they actually did. For example, for Ben Little, the agenda was to increase his assertiveness, yet any manifestations of increased assertiveness appeared to be either ignored, devalued, or reacted to with anger.

Table 10.3 Consistency or inconsistency, and the hidden or shared character of the foster parents' agenda and evaluations

Foster parents	Adolescent	Consistent agenda	Inconsistent agenda	Hidden agenda predominates	Explicit agenda predominates	Mix of hidden and open evaluation	Hidden evaluation predominates	Evaluation of placement agreed	Evaluation of placement not agreed
		3	4	5	6	7	8	9	10
Armstrong	Tim Larkin	*			*			*	
	Mark Robinson	*				*		*	
	Wayne Brett	*					*		
	Andy West	*			*			*	
	Tom Skipper	*			*			*	
	Paul Elliott (ii)	*					*		
Campbell	Wendy Bell	*			*				
Goldman	Kevin Flynn		*				*		
Hatton	Dawn Gibson		*			*		*	
	Christine Faber	*				*		*	
	Mandy Shepperd		*	*		*		*	
	Julie Piggett	*		*		*		*	
Harding	Paul Elliott (i)		*	*			*		
Henderson	Clare Dobson		*	*			*	*	
	Gina Fitzgerald		*				*	*	
	Diane White		*	*		*			*
Knight	Veronica Williams	*				*			*
Murphy	Rose Phillips	*				*		*	
	Frank Little	*				*			*
Page	Eddie Lewis		*				*		
Rushmoor	Vicky Jones	*			*			*	
Wilkinson	Lee Robinson	*					*		*
	Ben Little		*	*		*			*

Whether the foster parents' agenda was explicitly shared or hidden from the adolescent

In every case the foster parents' agenda showed a measure of explicitness; the contract meeting at the beginning of the placement ensured this. No instances of hidden agenda were identified in the placements studied retrospectively, although this might be attributed to the limitations of retrospective study. Instances of hidden agenda were identified in seven out of eleven prospective studies.

In each case the foster parents' hidden agenda became a major issue in the interaction between them and the adolescent. It seems as though what cannot be made explicit will be acted out in the interaction. For example, from the point when Clare Dobson declared herself pregnant and the Hendersons inwardly resolved that she must leave within three months, Clare's provocative behaviour escalated, bringing the placement to an end much sooner. The Knights privately hoped to direct Veronica Williams away from her plans to return to her family; Veronica engineered the two families into direct conflict and returned home. A similar pattern emerged in Mandy Shepperd's placement, when she ended the placement by going off on holiday with her previous foster parents, the only people in a long line of carers from whom the foster mother wished to divert her.

The evidence points towards inexplicit or hidden agenda constituting a powerful and unhelpful dynamic in a placement. Part of the skill for foster parents may well lie in identifying and finding ways of sharing those aspects of their agenda that they fear may not please the adolescent.

Agreement or disagreement in evaluation of success of placement

Finally one aspect of shared meanings between foster parents and adolescents is considered.

In thirteen placements there was a large measure of agreement between adolescents and foster parents about the success or failure of the placement and the nature of the change that had taken place (see Table 10.3, col. 9). In five of these there was agreement that the placement had been successful; in five that it had been partially successful; in three that it had been a failure. In five placements there was disagreement about the success or failure of the placement

159

(see Table 10.3, col. 10). In three of these the foster parents were very much less aware of success than the adolescents. In five placements, there was no evidence of the adolescent's evaluation of the placement. In each of these cases the foster parents regarded the placement as a failure, with either no change in the adolescent's functioning or a deterioration.

EVOLVING THEORY

In the earlier statement of the researcher's theoretical starting point, it was suggested that the therapeutic potential of the foster family depended on the relationship offering both continuity and the possibility of change. Continuity of relationship is only possible where there is a certain degree of overlap in the meaning that the adolescent and foster parents attribute to the placement and to their relationship. At the very least, foster parents need to be able to recognize and respect aspects of the adolescent's agenda, even if they also acknowledge that it differs from their own.

It has been further argued that a large measure of hidden agenda is liable to hinder reappraisal of self in relationship with others, whether the 'others' are the current foster parents or members of the adolescent's birth family. Whether the hidden agenda involves conflict or collusion, it promotes acting out of earlier patterns of behaviour within the relationship, rather than allowing these to be challenged or reflected upon. As long as this is happening, the adolescent is not able to operate in a truly autonomous manner in the present.

It seems important to look at the balance in the relationship between explicit meaning, agreed or debated, and inexplicit, unshared meanings, whether the latter conceal conflict or agreement. With this in mind, it is possible to arrange the placements in three groupings as in Table 10.4.

Group 1 (5 placements): those where there was a large measure of explicit meaning in the relationship

In these placements the foster parents' agenda was coherent and consistent, with little evidence of hidden agenda. All the adolescents remained in placement for the planned length of time (8–26 months). All agreed the placement had been a success, and all

Table 10.4 Placements grouped according to the balance of explicit meaning agreed or debated within the relationship and inexplicit, unshared meaning, which is collusive or conflicting

Name of foster parents	1 Relationships based predominantly on explicit meanings	2 Relationships based on a mixture of explicit and hidden meanings	3 Relationships based predominantly on hidden meanings
Armstrong	Tim Larkin Tom Skipper Andy West	Mark Robinson	Wayne Brett Paul Elliott (ii)
Campbell	Wendy Bell		
Harding			Paul Elliott (i)
Henderson		Diane White	Clare Dobson Gina Fitzgerald
Knight		Veronica Williams	
Murphy		Rose Phillips Frank Little	
Page			Eddie Lewis
Rushmoor	Vicky Jones		
Wilkinson		Lee Robinson Ben Little	
Hatton		Dawn Dibson Mandy Shepperd Christine Faber Julie Piggett	
Goldman			Kevin Flynn
	5 placements	11 placements	7 placements

remained in contact with each other after the placement ended. Four of these placements were in group 4 of Table 10.2; that is, the adolescents were perceived by their foster parents to have made progress during the placement. The relationships in these placements could be considered mutually satisfying. The evidence points to such a relationship helping the reparative process.

Group 2 (11 placements): those where there was a mix of explicit meaning and hidden meaning in the relationship

In seven of these the foster parents' agenda was consistent, but in two cases there was also hidden agenda. In four placements the foster parents' agenda was inconsistent, in three of these four there was also hidden agenda. Seven of these placements disrupted. Placements lasted between 3½–26 months. Six agreed their evaluation of the placement; in five cases that it had been at least partially successful, and in one case that it had been a failure. Of the five where there was disagreement in their evaluation of the placement it was in the direction of adolescents being more positive and foster parents negative. In these it seems that the foster parents had not been able to keep in touch with or go along with the adolescents' agenda or goals for the placement. Six kept in touch with the adolescents after the placement ended.

Ten of these placements were in groups 2 or 3 of Table 10.2; that is, their foster parents' perceptions of them were mixed. The relationships in these placements might be described as ambiguous but, with one exception, at least partially satisfying.

Group 3 (7 placements): those where there was little shared meaning and a large measure of hidden agenda in the relationship

Placements in this group lasted between 3½–12 months. All either agreed the placement had been a failure, or the foster parents thought so and there was no evaluation from the adolescents. None remained in contact with each other when the placement ended.

Four of these placements were in group 1 of Table 10.2; that is, the adolescents were perceived by their foster parents as destructive, victims of circumstances, and unmotivated for family placement. The relationship in these placements might be described as mutually unsatisfying. The evidence points to such a relationship hindering the reparative process.

CONCLUSION

Movement towards autonomy, defined as the ability to accurately appraise self in relationships and to judge when it is appropriate to call on the help of other trusted people, is put forward as the preferred outcome of foster placement of difficult adolescents. For this to be achieved foster parents need to be emotionally available to the adolescent placed with them. This is the essential condition if the adolescents are to experience the foster parents as a secure base from which to explore and establish themselves in the adult world outside the foster family.

In this paper criteria have been identified for judging the quality of relationship offered by the foster parents to the adolescent in their care. These are:

1. The extent to which the foster parents' agenda for the placement overlaps with the purposes identified as important to the adolescent.
2. The extent to which the foster parents' agenda is set at a level likely to be attainable by an adolescent in a time-limited placement.
3. The extent to which the foster parents' agenda is consistent through the placement.
4. The extent to which the foster parents' agenda is shared openly and explicitly with the adolescent, whether or not this leads to agreement or disagreement about the purposes of the placement.

When these criteria are fulfilled, the relationship offered by foster parents during the placement will have the potential for being experienced as a secure base for exploration. Additionally, the placement is more likely to run for its planned course, and foster parents and adolescent to continue to keep in touch with each other once it ends.

It follows from this that the quality of life experienced by foster parents is closely bound up with their potential for improving the quality of life for difficult adolescents in care. Successful placements tend to be those with shared goals and a shared sense of progress and achievement. One practice implication is that social workers should pay particular attention to placements where foster parents have more doubts about the value of what they are doing than does the adolescent. This may involve helping foster parents towards a more realistic agenda for the placement and encouraging more open sharing and feedback between them and the adolescent, even at the risk of conflict. It is vitally important to reassure foster parents of their value to adolescents in care, especially when adolescents have difficulty conveying this themselves.

REFERENCES

Bowlby, J. (1969) *Attachment and Loss: vol. 1 Attachment*, London: Hogarth Press and the Institute of Psycho-analysis.

Bowlby, J. (1973) *Attachment and Loss: vol. 2 Separation; Anxiety and Anger*, London: Hogarth Press and the Institute of Psycho-analysis.

Bowlby, J. (1979) 'Self-reliance and some conditions that promote it', in J. Bowlby, *The Making and Breaking of Affectional Bonds*, London: Tavistock, pp. 103–25.

Brown, G. W. and Harris, T. O. (1978) *Social Origins of Depression*, London: Tavistock.

Downes, C. (1986) 'The reparative potential of foster family interaction: difficult adolescents in time-limited placements', unpublished D.Phil. thesis, University of York.

Downes, C. (1988) 'Foster families for adolescents: the healing potential of time-limited placements', *British Journal of Social Work* 18:473–87.

Henderson, S. (1982) 'The significance of social relationships in the etiology of neurosis', in C. M. Parkes and J. Stevenson-Hinde (eds) *The Place of Attachment in Human Behaviour*, London: Tavistock.

Parkes, C. M. (1982) 'Attachment and the prevention of mental disorders', in C. M. Parkes and J. Stevenson-Hinde (eds) *The Place of Attachment in Human Behaviour*, London: Tavistock.

Weiss, R. S. (1982) 'Attachment in adult life', in C. M. Parkes and J. Stevenson-Hinde (eds) *The Place of Attachment in Human Behaviour*, London: Tavistock.

Chapter Eleven

CHOICE AND SELF-DETERMINATION AS ASPECTS OF QUALITY OF LIFE IN PRIVATE SECTOR HOMES

ANNE CORDEN

A CHANGING PATTERN OF PROVISION

It is now 25 years since Townsend's harrowing account of institutional life for elderly people (Townsend 1962). The radical change in policy towards residential provision for elderly people heralded by the 1948 National Assistance Act, moving towards smaller, more homely units of local authority residential care, was implemented only slowly. Townsend had found in 1960 that 'the mainstay of local authority residential services for the handicapped and aged' (1962:29) was still the old workhouse building. Of the local authority homes visited, one third offered very bad facilities, and another third not much better. His account of the quality of the residents' lives makes sad reading.

Throughout the 1950s and 1960s general agreement that elderly people should stay at home as long as possible was based not only on concern for their welfare, but also on considerations of the financial burden on the community of maintaining extensive hospital and residential provision (Sheldon 1984). Such views fitted in with current assumptions about the obligations of the family (Means and Smith 1985). Despite a shift in policy emphasis from institution to community, there was little corresponding shift in resources. Demographic pressures from an ageing population (Wicks 1982) contributed to increasing demand for community-based services – home helps, meals on wheels, etc. Increasingly, voluntary organizations were drawn in to cope with the shortfall in statutory services. Failure to expand community services meant that the need for residential care continued. In 1976, the DHSS acknowledged that 'there will still be many old people for whom there is no alternative to residential care' (DHSS 1976a).

The pattern of residential provision began to change. Public sector provision began to level off, and NHS geriatric provision to fall. A dynamic increase in the number of places for elderly people in private homes began. There has always been a private sector. Townsend estimated that about a tenth of residents of pensionable age in residential institutions were in private homes. But by 1979, numbers of elderly people in private homes had overtaken those in the voluntary sector, and rapid expansion in the numbers of private nursing homes had begun. Currently more than half of all long term residential care for elderly people is provided by the private and voluntary sectors (Laing and Buisson 1991).

RESEARCH ON INSTITUTIONS FOR ELDERLY PEOPLE

Townsend had found striking variation in the facilities, management and staffing in the private homes, but considered more than one third to be very poor. Has the expansion in the market improved the quality of life in the private sector?

There has been no lack of critics of conditions in the private sector: in the media (Smith 1986), among trade unionists representing NHS workers (Holmes 1986), and in the medical profession (Primrose 1987). The controversy is heightened by the concern that many elderly residents are supported by public funds, via income support (previously supplementary benefit). Currently, more than half of those in private and voluntary residential care and nursing homes are income support claimants (Laing and Buisson 1991). The growth in supplementary benefit expenditure on fees was a major concern within DHSS throughout the 1980s. Among the issues addressed by two joint central/local government working parties were the quality of service for publicly funded residents in the independent sector, and whether the care provided matched their needs and represented value for money (Scott-Whyte 1985:10).

Despite the expansion in the private sector, proper evidence of the quality of life in these homes is thin on the ground. Only a few homes approach such extremes of poor quality that they are exposed in the media, or have their registration withdrawn. As Day and Klein point out 'the real challenge lies in defining bench marks which allow us to know as a matter of routine, and in good time, that care is being provided to acceptable standards, and to assess changes over time' (Day and Klein 1987:385). This has proved fairly difficult.

The problems of looking at quality of life in institutions are not confined to the private sector. The first problem, the complexity of the task, is general to research in all institutional settings. Each resident's quality of life will depend on a multiplicity of components. A model of influences on consumer satisfaction in a residential setting, developed for a study in local authority homes, identified various characteristics of the physical environment, the resident mix, and the institutional environment which interact to produce different impacts on each resident according to his or her background, characteristics, and preferences (Willcocks *et al.* 1982). Investigation of all these dimensions requires a variety of research techniques.

A second problem is the infirmity of many residents. A feasibility study used to develop survey measures of the quality of life of elderly people in residential care (Peace *et al.* 1979) found many difficulties in seeking the experiences of very old and infirm residents. A number could not communicate at all; residents found interviews too long and tiring; they did not understand scales and frequently felt unable to criticize aspects of the home in which they were to spend the remaining part of their lives. Wilkin, attempting to interview elderly residents in Part III homes, also found constraints in response due to the infirmity of residents, and the institutional context (Wilkin and Hughes 1987). Challis and Bartlett tried an observational and listening approach rather than direct questioning but found it difficult to get beyond an overwhelming undercurrent of patients' sadness (Challis and Bartlett 1987, 1988). Stock Whitaker (1988), talking to residents in Part III homes, has tried yet another approach based on sentence completion techniques. There is room for much development in methodology in eliciting the attitudes and experiences of very frail elderly people.

A third problem is identified by Day and Klein (1987). They argue that there are no agreed measures of standards and quality of care. The recommendations of *Home Life* (1984) and the Handbook for Health Authorities (1985) provide assistance in fulfilling the requirements of the Registered Homes Act 1984. However, interpretations of adequate standards show marked differences between authorities, making comparison and assessment very difficult.

These difficulties are not peculiar to the private sector, but one problem that may indeed be more significant in the private sector is that of access. The researcher enters a private home by invitation only. Regulating authorities may support research and recommend participation, but have little real leverage in evoking cooperation. Similarly, associations of home owners can encourage members to participate in research, but are prepared to recommend non-cooperation where they feel this appropriate. Many private homes are not only an institutional setting for residents but the owner's private domestic home as well, and questions asked in research can intrude on personal philosophies, self images, family dynamics and financial situations. With extensive duties the proprietor may give low priority to time-consuming research instruments or interviews. Ernst and Whinney found difficulty in obtaining response to a survey in a national research study (Ernst and Whinney 1986). On a smaller scale, questionnaires sent to private homes in North Wales evoked low response rates, considered to be due to reluctance to divulge confidential information, and the workload involved in completion (Humphreys and Kassab 1986).

Finally, there may be particular problems in the nursing home sector. It is not clear how nursing homes fit into the general philosophies of residential care. They are registered and inspected by health authority personnel with medical and nursing backgrounds, but there is no model of good practice within most health authorities since only three have an experimental NHS nursing home. Is the quality of life to be assessed in comparison with a geriatric ward, using a medical model and corresponding emphasis on delivery of nursing care, or should comparison be made with the residential model, with an added medical input? The latter option may be problematic because residential and nursing regimes are so different, as are the aims and expertise of those professionals who deliver and regulate care in the two sectors. The emphasis in delivery of nursing services is often the quality of care, but this does not equate with quality of life.

In view of the complexity of the task, and apparent difficulties, it is perhaps not surprising that there has been only one major comprehensive study of residential life in private homes for elderly people that included the attitudes and preferences of the residents themselves (Weaver et al. 1985). Most other researchers have made their own observations, focusing on just one or a few contributory aspects to life, for example the dependency of residents (Wade et al. 1983; Primrose and Capewell 1986); the physical environment and characteristics of staff and proprietors (Bartlett and Challis 1986); the facilities available, and the corresponding charges (Judge 1984). This chapter also reports findings at this level – observations of a particular aspect of quality of life, from a small scale local study, to contribute to the general picture of the provision made by private care for elderly people.

The focus of interest in this paper is the amount of choice available to people entering the private sector, and their scope for determining and controlling the parameters of their lives. This focus has been chosen because one of the main arguments used by those who supported the development of private care using supplementary benefit was that the private sector increases the choice available to elderly people, and provides opportunities for self-determination without the direction and paternalism of professional advisors and gatekeepers. The importance of maintaining choice and independence is a recurrent theme in the psychology of ageing (Baltes and Baltes 1986) and in the philosophy of residential care (DHSS 1976; Brearley 1977; *Home Life* 1984). Research conducted in the Social Policy Research Unit at the University of York provided an opportunity to investigate the reality of the apparent choice opened up by the availability of supplementary benefit.

RESEARCH ON RESIDENTIAL CARE AND NURSING HOMES IN NORTH YORKSHIRE

The details of the research project are described elsewhere (SPRU 1985). Briefly, the study monitored the effects of changes in supplementary benefit regulations for elderly people in, or seeking places in, private and voluntary residential and nursing home care in two local areas over a period of two and a half years. A variety of statistical and qualitative techniques were used. The following discussion draws on findings from a postal survey of all proprietors in North Yorkshire at the end of 1985; in-depth interviews with a sample of 40 proprietors of residential and nursing homes; and interviews with key personnel in the five health authorities, and the social services department covering North Yorkshire.

It was not possible in this study to ask elderly people what choice they exercised in entering a home. Weaver *et al.* (1985) found that those residents who had best been able to come to terms with life in a private residential home were those who had exercised some degree of control in entering care. Only 26 per cent of that sample reported having had a choice of home. Twenty-two per cent said their admission was the result of 'unsolicited arrangements' made by a third party. Real choice between entering a home and continuing to cope in the community is constrained by many circumstances of health and housing, availability of potential carers, and alternative packages of care. Other research has addressed whether elderly people need to go into residential homes (Gibbs and Bradshaw 1987). This paper presents the perspective for an elderly person who had decided there was no alternative to institutional care, and wanted a suitable place in North Yorkshire.

CHOICE OF FACILITIES IN NORTH YORKSHIRE

At the time of the survey there were 47 local authority Part III homes in North Yorkshire. In the same area there were 178 private and voluntary residential homes for elderly people. Local people seeking places may look to a smaller area. To give a more realistic impression, in the environs of York there were 13 Part III facilities, with a further 9 private residential homes and 7 private nursing homes. Moreover, any choice in size of establishment, towards a smaller, more domestic environment, lay almost entirely within the private and voluntary sector. All except two of the Part III homes around York had 40 or more residents whereas nearly one half of the private and voluntary residential homes in North Yorkshire had fewer than 10 residents. Very few North Yorkshire nursing homes had more than 30 patients at that time.

So, choice for a resident in York, Scarborough or Harrogate was certainly extended by the private sector, both in terms of number of homes and towards smaller, more homely settings. There is a different perspective from more rural areas, since private homes cluster round the larger towns. Although the percentage of the population aged over 60 years in the Hambleton/Richmond area of the county was almost as high as in the York area, and had been growing at twice the rate in the last fifteen years, much of this part of the county had no nursing homes and only two residential homes. An elderly person here would have to look further afield, towards Harrogate or Skipton. For an elderly person seeking to move into the county to be near relatives, choice would lie only in the independent sector, but again heavily concentrated around the main towns. Half the private nursing homes in North Yorkshire were in Harrogate and environs.

Further restriction on choice operates through the availability of vacancies. Detailed interviews in early 1987 with proprietors of 20 private nursing homes showed that half had no vacancies, and six of these had long waiting lists. Again, the picture was variable according to locality. All four nursing homes in the western area of the county had waiting lists. Only one home among four visited in the Scarborough/east coast area had a vacancy. Most of the vacancies were in Harrogate and the surrounding area, with a few in the York environs. There were only three vacancies in single rooms among the 20 nursing homes. All other vacant beds were in double or multi-bedded rooms, which further restricted access by gender. The characteristics of the room may impose further restrictions on choice. Two nursing homes had some bedrooms that could only accommodate mobile people, since they were up staircases with no lifts. Patients who needed access to hoists, or particular medical apparatus would be further restricted to particular rooms in several homes.

Finding a vacancy is no guarantee of a place. Nursing homes are registered to accept patients with particular needs, and on subsequent inspection visits the health authority monitors whether the home is taking patients for whom it is properly equipped to care. However, even within this authorization most owners of nursing homes interviewed in 1987 were operating careful gatekeeping procedures. This was because some patients need particularly high levels of attention, while some are disruptive or prone to upsetting other patients. One proprietor did not accept men, while another operated a gender quotient of one-third men. In most nursing homes women outnumber men by four to one, so in the latter home there was a longer waiting list for women. Only three proprietors were prepared to consider all people, however dependent. The others considered some patients unacceptable. These could include people who wandered, those with severe dementia, aggressive or obese people. Ambulant confused men were particularly unwelcome, and patients known to be destructive to furnishings were avoided. Proprietors who would consider severely confused or aggressive people would often only have one at a time.

The final restriction on choice may be the level of fees. At the time of this study more than half the residents in the independent sector depended on supplementary benefit. The regulations were complex, but the current scheme was one of national limits to the amount of supplementary benefit that might be paid, according to the type of care received. For example, at the time of the survey (1987) an elderly person who was eligible for supplementary benefit could claim up to £120 per week towards fees for residential care, or £170 in a nursing home, with an additional personal allowance of £8.95. If weekly fees were higher than these levels, supplementary benefit claimants had to look to other resources to make up the difference.

This situation was examined in 1985, on the basis of postal replies from 54 nursing homes in North Yorkshire. When the supplementary benefit limit was £170 weekly for elderly people in nursing homes, only 13 homes were offering accommodation in single rooms at or below this limit when vacancies occurred. Rather more, 30 out of 54, were offering shared accommodation within this limit. The pattern was variable. In the east coast area, and the west of the county, only one quarter of homes offered no accommodation at all at or below the supplementary benefit limit. The proportion rose to 45 per cent in the Harrogate area, and in the York area nearly 60 per cent of nursing homes were charging fees for all rooms above the limit. People dependent on supplementary benefit, seeking a single room in the Harrogate area, could only consider 18 per cent of homes unless they used their personal allowance for fees. Similar people seeking single rooms in the Scarborough area could consider half the nursing homes.

There was a similar picture in the residential sector. In Scarborough, 95 per cent of the residential care homes for elderly people quoted basic weekly charges at or below the supplementary benefit limit; indeed 65 per cent offered single rooms at this rate, if they had a vacancy. In the York area, by contrast, only 30 per cent quoted charges within the limit, and only 2 of the 17 homes in the area covered by the York supplementary benefit office could offer single room accommodation at this rate.

These findings suggest that real choice is highly restricted by availability of vacancies, proprietors' gatekeeping procedures and financial accessibility. Those wanting choice of a particular location in the county, or single rooms, are further restricted. Limited knowledge may further restrict choice. It is not known how much information applicants gather, but there are indications that it may be very little. The avenues for seeking such information are limited. Registration authorities in North Yorkshire issue lists of registered homes in their area of authority. These are limited to names of proprietors, addresses and telephone numbers of homes, number of places and types of resident authorized.

Only a small proportion of homes advertise. Many elderly people use the evening paper as a familiar source of local knowledge, but few homes maintain advertising space here once well established. Of the 20 nursing homes studied 12 had taken no advertising initiative apart from Yellow Pages listings. One quarter had no brochure or printed material available to send out. Only 6 of the 15 brochures that were available from this sample were designed to include current fees.

All proprietors reported encouraging elderly people or relatives to visit before moving in, but said this was often difficult to arrange. Many elderly people entered their homes without visiting them first or meeting the person in charge. At the time of this study a policy directive to North Yorkshire social workers restricted the advice they might give to people seeking a place in the private sector. National charities for the welfare of elderly people produce general information and advice about choosing a home, and local offices of Age Concern in North Yorkshire maintain a certain amount of factual information about local homes. Their policy is not to recommend homes but to encourage people to visit themselves, and transport can be made available for this.

Indications from this research are that opportunities for real choice of home are limited. Such findings support those of Weaver *et al.* when 61 per cent of residents interviewed in private homes 'failed to report having made a positive choice based on even the most arbitrary of criteria' (Weaver *et al.* 1985:31) and less than two in five had visited before admission. North Yorkshire proprietors said it was possible for residents to come for a trial period, but this appeared to be of little real significance in extending choice. It was rare for patients to leave nursing homes after arrival. A few occasions were recalled when patients had been asked to leave because of difficult behaviour. Two nursing homes had established special arrangements with a local psychogeriatric hospital whereby they took dementing patients on a trial basis. However this was to see if proprietors could cope, rather than whether patients liked the home.

In questioning how far the private sector increases choice we do not know what extent of choice elderly people would like, nor how far and on what dimensions they actually exercise choice. We do not know the extent of their knowledge about the options available.

Evidence presented suggests that the range of options may be small, and knowledge about such options even smaller.

OPPORTUNITIES FOR SELF-DETERMINATION

The research findings also challenged the assumption that the private sector increases opportunities for self-determination, and control of their own lives for elderly people. This research did not address whether elderly people had any control over whether they went into a home but points to what can happen once they arrive.

Those who supported the availability of supplementary benefit for people in private care argued that, by having access to the necessary finance, an elderly person was better able to decide the type of care best suited to her needs. People with limited income then had equal opportunities for the type of control available to their wealthier peers. The right of wealthier people to this type of self-determination was strongly defended by the private sector itself. 'People paying for their own care should always have the right to choose the type of care they feel suits their needs ...' (Stanniland 1987). However, it is acknowledged that such self-determination may have inherent dangers, as well as opportunities. People may move into institutional care before they need it. Although one study suggested that this may not be such a large problem as had been anticipated (Gibbs and Bradshaw 1987), it has now been agreed that some assessment of needs to ensure appropriate placement is desirable, at least for those supported by public funds.

The atmosphere, regime, and quality of care of a home depend largely on the characteristics and attitudes of the managers. In a study of 118 private residential homes in Devon in 1984, one quarter of proprietors anticipated remaining in business only a short time (Phillips and Vincent 1986). The authors suggested that 'the potential for continuing rapid turnover of ownership in the sector should be a cause for concern for policy makers and for the professionals involved in care for the elderly' (Phillips and Vincent 1986:170). Our results showed that of those North Yorkshire homes established in January 1986, 21 per cent had undergone a change in ownership by mid-1987. Residents were not always told about impending changes in ownership until contracts were signed, or a new owner introduced himself! The subsequent changes in regime may not have been anticipated by residents and may not have been welcome.

Residents may also experience a major change in the size of the home or the resident mix. A small homely atmosphere may well have been promoted when the home opened, but many proprietors told us that subsequent expansion was essential for economic viability. Of the 20 nursing homes studied 11 had already extended their premises to enlarge their capacity, and 6 of those not yet extended were planning to do so in the coming year. The environment can be altered considerably by such developments. A small four-bedded home had rapidly been extended into next door premises to accommodate 14 patients. A compact town house with 30 patients had undergone substantial redevelopment, incorporating long corridors for wandering about, with eventual capacity for 42 patients.

Similarly, current residents have little control over the general resident mix. Some proprietors do make considerable efforts to find compatible people to share rooms. Similarly, a patient who upsets others may eventually be asked to leave, or efforts made to isolate him or her to a particular room. To this extent, some patients are able to exercise some influence. But some decisions about the resident mix are unlikely to be referred to current residents for consideration. For example, a change in registration may introduce a different proportion of dementing people. Do current residents find such changes unwelcome? A move towards dual registration might be experienced as a real advantage. The point made is that the environment can change very quickly, away from original expectations, with little opportunity for control by the resident.

Constraints on self-determination considered so far affect all residents, whether privately or publicly funded. Further constraints and potential insecurities were identified for residents dependent on supplementary benefit. Since 1983 there was a series of major adjustments to the regulations governing payment of supplementary benefit to people in the independent sector, and changes in the amounts of money that might be claimed. Proprietors responded to these changes. Although there was some partial protection for long-term residents, more recent entrants and people seeking places were certainly affected. Whereas proprietors had been prepared to hold down charges for established patients whose supplementary benefit entitlement did not meet current fees, most insisted on full rates from new entrants, and some had to use their personal allowance to meet basic fees. Consequently, there was inadequate money for patients' clothing. A large proportion of proprietors interviewed relied on jumble sales, or the clothing of patients who had died. Others insisted on top-ups from relatives, and sometimes approached charities.

The research did not address how far elderly people want to control their lives. Many of our findings, however, made us reflect on the general assumption that the private sector offers increased opportunities for self-determination. We suggest that for very frail and vulnerable members of society, there can only be self-determination if there are also opportunities for representation and advocacy. Proprietors of private homes are accountable to the registration authorities for the conditions in their homes and the quality of care. Although the resident has some protection via this regulation process, he or she can still be very isolated. Most patients in private nursing homes are very old – at least 64 per cent of those claiming supplementary benefit in North Yorkshire were over 80. Some are very confused; immobile and unable to communicate. Many have no immediate relatives; where they do have spouses, or children, these are often frail pensioners themselves. At this stage, a need for self-determination has to be balanced against a need for responsible, caring advocacy, representation, and accountability of those responsible. It was rare in North Yorkshire in the 1980s for local authority social workers to maintain links with elderly people in the private sector; health authorities and proprietors reported that GPs were increasingly anxious about the amount of time they could give to these patients; the appointee system, whereby elderly people's supplementary benefit is managed for them, appeared to be in need of reexamination; access to some basic NHS facilities such as chiropody and physiotherapy was much reduced. Factors like this suggested that the potential opportunity for self-determination in the private sector could actually result in increased isolation and dependency.

It has not been the aim in this chapter to criticize the quality of life in the private sector. We were, on many occasions, impressed by proprietors' attitudes and efforts made on behalf of their residents. We saw also things that concerned us. However, the private sector does not have a monopoly of problems – there are disadvantages of institutions which are general to all such environments, whether run for profit, or through charity, or public administration. The point made is that there is little well-founded evidence of the relative importance of aspects we assume contribute to the quality of life for elderly people in institutions. Research techniques on this topic are still to be developed; the consumer's voice has hardly made any contribution to this debate, and we need to look beyond the rhetoric of enthusiasm for a particular policy, for the real evidence of what is being provided.

REFERENCES

Baltes, M. and Baltes, P. (eds) (1986) *The Psychology of Control and Ageing*, New Jersey: Lawrence Erlbaum.

Bartlett, H. and Challis, L. (1986) *Private Nursing Homes for the Elderly*, Working Paper no. 3, Centre for the Analysis of Social Policy, University of Bath.

Brearley, C. P. (1977) *Residential Work with the Elderly*, London: Routledge & Kegan Paul.

Challis, L. and Bartlett, H. (1987, 1988) *Old and Ill, Private Nursing Homes for Elderly People* , Age Concern, Institute of Gerontology Research Paper no. 1.

Day, P. and Klein, R. (1987) 'Quality of institutional care and the elderly: policy issues and options', *British Medical Journal* 294 (February).

DHSS (1976a) *Priorities for Health and Personal Social Services in England*, HMSO, p. 42.

DHSS (1976b) *A Lifestyle for the Elderly*, London: HMSO.

Ernst and Whinney (1986) *Survey of Private and Voluntary Residential and Nursing Homes*, London: DHSS.

Firth, J. (1987) *Public Support for Residential Care*, Report of a joint central and local government working party, London: DHSS.

Gibbs, I. and Bradshaw, J. (1987) 'Needs must fit', *Social Services Insight* 2 (30) (July).

Handbook for Health Authorities (1985) *Registration and Inspection of Nursing Homes*, National Association of Health Authorities in England and Wales.

Holmes, B./NUPE (1986) *The Realities of Home Life, NUPE/Economic Development Committee of West Midlands CC.*

Home Life: A Code of Practice for Residential Care (1984) London: Centre for Policy on Ageing.

Humphreys, H. and Kassab, J. (1986) 'An investigation into private sector nursing and residential home care for the elderly in North Wales', *Journal of the Royal College of General Practitioners* 36 (November).

Judge, K. (1984) *Why Do Private Residential Care Home Charges Vary?* PSSRU, University of Kent.

Laing and Buisson (1991) *Care of Elderly People*, Market Survey 1991–92, London: Laing and Buisson Publications Ltd.

Means, R. and Smith, R. (1985) *The Development of Welfare Services for Elderly People*, London: Croom Helm, pp. 240–3.

OPCS (1971–86) Annual population estimates.

Pearce, S., Hall, J., and Hamblin, G. (1979) *The Quality of Life of the Elderly in Residential Care: A Feasibility Study of the Development of Survey Measures*, Research Report no. 1, Survey Research Unit, Polytechnic of North London.

Phillips, D. and Vincent, J. (1986) 'Private residential accommodation for the elderly: geographical aspects of developments in Devon', *Trans. Inst. Br. Geogr.* 11:155–73.

Primrose, W. (1987) 'General Practitioners and Registered Nursing Homes in Edinburgh', *Health Bulletin* 45 (2) March.

Primrose, W. and Capewell, A. (1986) 'A survey of registered nursing homes in Edinburgh', *Journal of the Royal College of General Practitioners* 36 (March).

Rossiter, C. and Wicks, M. (1982) *Crisis or Challenge, Family Care, Elderly People and Social Policy*, Occasional Paper no. 8, London: Study Commission on the Family.

Scott-Whyte, S. (1985) *Supplementary Benefit and Residential Care*, Report of a joint central and local government working party, London: DHSS.

Sheldon, J. H. (1954) 'The social philosophy of old age', in *Old Age in the Modern World*, Report of the Third Congress of the International Association of Gerontology, London.

Smith, A. (1986) 'Society tomorrow', *Guardian*, 12 November.

SPRU (1985) 'Proposal for a study to monitor the impact of the new supplementary benefit board and lodging regulations on elderly people in private and voluntary residential care and nursing homes', DHSS Working Paper 257, Social Policy Research Unit, University of York.

Stanniland, P. (1987) *Nursing Home Care*, Registered Nursing Home Association 1987.

Stock Whitaker, D. (1987) Presentation at the Third Annual Conference on Research into Practice, Joint University Council/British Association of Social Workers.

Townsend, P. (1962) *The Last Refuge*, London: Routledge & Kegan Paul.

Wade, B., Sawyer, L., and Bell, J. (1983) *Dependency with Dignity*, Occasional Papers on Social Administration no. 68, Bedford Square Press/NCVO.

Weaver, T., Willcocks, D., and Kellaher, L. (1985) *The Business of Care: A Study of Private Residential Homes for Old People*, CESSA Report no. 1, Polytechnic of North London.

Wilkin, D. and Hughes, B. (1987) 'Residential care of elderly people: the consumers' views', *Ageing and Society* 7.

Willcocks, D., Pearce, S., and Kellaher, L. and with Ring, L. (1982) *The Residential Life of Old People: A Study in 100 Local Authority Homes*, Research Report no. 12, Survey Research Unit, Polytechnic of North London.

Chapter Twelve

TESTING TOWNSEND
Exploring living standards using secondary data analysis [1]
SANDRA HUTTON

Townsend (1979) defined poverty in terms of relative deprivation and controversially illustrated how such a concept could be made operational by developing a deprivation index. Since then little empirical work has been done to follow up and replicate his results, and this paper describes the first stages of such a study. Information from the Family Expenditure Survey (FES) and the General Household Survey (GHS) is used here to develop a measure of the standard of living of the breadth required by such a definition of poverty, and to investigate how this measure varies with income. The paper briefly outlines Townsend's ideas, reviews the subsequent discussion of his work and then goes on to consider the data available in the FES and GHS and discusses their adequacy as inputs to measures of standards of living. Finally some initial analyses of possible indicators of standards of living will be illustrated with results for one family type.

TOWNSEND'S IDEAS

Townsend proposed that 'poverty can be defined objectively and applied consistently only in terms of relative deprivation' (Townsend 1979). Prior to this, early empirical studies on the measure of poverty had defined poverty in narrow 'absolute' or 'subsistence' terms. For example, Rowntree defined people as being in primary poverty if 'total earnings are insufficient to obtain the minimum necessaries for the maintenance of merely physical efficiency' (Rowntree 1901:117). The comparison of resources and needs continues to be the basis for the measurement of poverty but the use of earnings as the measure of resources and of physical efficiency as the measure of

179

needs have long been thought of as too restrictive.

In the post-war studies of poverty other measures of resources were used: Abel-Smith and Townsend pioneered the use of the FES for the measurement of poverty and used total expenditure as a better measure of command over resources than merely earnings or even current total income (Abel-Smith and Townsend 1965). Other later studies have also used expenditure as well as income, but in the main income is still used as the measure of resources although including as far as possible income from all sources (Fiegehen, Lansley, and Smith 1977; Bradshaw, Cooke, and Godfrey 1984).

For the measurement of needs, the National Assistance and later the supplementary benefit scale rates have provided a convenient base. So although blurred by subsequent changes, the origins of these rates can be traced back through Beveridge to the very narrow definition of needs based on subsistence criteria. Also, what these rates really provided for in terms of needs is not at all clear.

What was new about what Townsend proposed? He suggested new ways of measurement of both resources and needs. He broadened the definition of resources to include 'all types of resources, public and private, which are distributed unequally in society and which contribute towards actual standards of living' (1979:60). His broader definition of needs, however, represented a bigger break with what had gone before – he stated people needed resources 'to obtain the type of diet, participate in the activities and have the living conditions and amenities which are customary or at least widely encouraged or approved in the societies to which they belong' (1979:30). Those in poverty are those whose resources are 'so seriously below those commanded by the average individual or family that they are, in effect, *excluded* from ordinary living patterns, customs and activities' (1979:30). He went on to hypothesize that 'as resources for any individual or family are diminished, there is a point at which there occurs a sudden withdrawal from participation in the customs and activities sanctioned by the culture. The point at which withdrawal escalates disproportionately to falling resources could be defined as the poverty line'. Thus his definition of poverty was behavioural and descriptive, with little moral connotation.

To test this hypothesis he undertook a detailed study of people's style of living and their resources. His survey of 2,000 households in 1968–9 asked for information on diet, clothing, fuel and light, home amenities, housing and housing facilities, the immediate environment of the home, the characteristics, security, general conditions and welfare benefits of work, family support, recreation, education, health, and social relations. He derived 60 indicators of deprivation – for example, lacking an amenity or not participating in an activity. A score for different forms of deprivation was added up – the higher the score, the greater the deprivation and a summary deprivation index was defined. This index was correlated with income and he tentatively suggested that a threshold existed such that at incomes near 150 per cent of the supplementary benefit scale rates deprivation significantly increased.

AFTER TOWNSEND – THE DEBATE AND FURTHER RESEARCH

After the publication of Townsend's study in 1979, Piachaud claimed that the index is not the objective measure sought and that it is implausible that a threshold should exist given two factors, that styles of living are diverse and that poverty is relative (Piachaud 1981). He also doubted the justification of using such a threshold to define poverty saying 'Poverty carries with it an implication and moral imperative that something should be done about it. Its definition is a value judgement and should be clearly seen to be so no matter how carefully styles of life are measured and indices computed' (Piachaud 1981:421).

Mack and Lansley in their 1985 survey made explicit the value judgements by asking a sample survey of 1,000 people which of 33 items they would regard as necessary and which all adults/families should be able to afford and which they should not have to do without (Mack and Lansley 1985). They defined as poor those who lacked three or more of the 14 items which the largest majority agreed to be necessities. Critics identified two problems with this approach: (a) if these items are really necessities, then lacking *one* should be defined as poverty; and (b) many who lacked 'necessities' so defined could afford non-necessities – should they also be called poor? (Ashton 1984; Piachaud 1987).

Sen makes the link between the measurement of poverty to the measurement of living standards:

The identification of the poor is an exercise in which the focus is on the minimum living conditions but the same approach can of course be used to rank the overall living standards of different persons and groups.

(Sen 1987:31)

The approach he suggests should be through the concept of capabilities to achieve certain living conditions and not through ideas of opulence, commodities, or utilities.

He also emphasizes that diversity is 'part of the traditional picture of living standard ... we must not sacrifice all the richness of the idea ... to get something nicely neat and agreeably simple' (Sen 1987:2). There is room for choice. This plea is also found in Atkinson's writings, which have particular relevance to the data-based approach used in this work. He suggests that the ability and desire to measure standards of living has been made possible by the fast development of computer technology and proposes that it should be possible to select one's own measure from a database. He also highlights the role of unobservable variables such as the distribution of income within the family and the level of consumption rather than consumer expenditure and the importance of choosing the correct unit of measurement (Atkinson 1974, 1984).

Townsend has also returned to the field with a survey of multiple deprivation in the London labour market 1985–6. He distinguishes between material and social deprivation and again affirms that the definition should be objective – it should comprise conditions, relationships, and behaviour rather than attitudes and beliefs (Townsend 1987).

CONTEXT OF THE PRESENT STUDY

Currently, the level of supplementary benefit (SB) is commonly used as the demarcation of poverty. The main advantage of this is that it represents the 'minimum standard of living that the government considers necessary at a particular time' (Atkinson 1974:48). Neither the standard of living allowed by the SB levels nor how this might relate to the standard of living enjoyed by the rest of the population is currently known (though see Bradshaw and Morgan 1987). If a relative definition of poverty is adopted, a generally accepted proposition now, the use of the current rates of benefit as a basis for the measurement of standards of living 'without any examination of the standard of living they represent amounts to a circular procedure' (Nicolson 1979:61). Thus there is a need to measure the standards of living over a range of incomes and within a broader context than Townsend's deprivation index. The aim of the study, of which this paper describes the first stages, is to develop further the empirical analysis of the concept of poverty which includes not only what people lack materially but also the extent to which they are socially excluded by their lack of resources. The key element in this is the measurement of living standards – defined as both having and doing – and the relationship between living standards and income. The first stage is thus a descriptive analysis of the living standards of families at different income levels and some results from this stage of the study are described below. The study aims to link the information from two large national surveys, the Family Expenditure Survey and the General Household Survey. The use of the FES in a measure of standards of living follows a long tradition (Bradshaw, Cooke, and Godfrey 1984; Fiegehen, Lansley, and Smith 1987). Expenditure itself is a narrow measure of living standards – accumulation of goods, proximity to work and leisure, for example, may mean that living standards are not what expenditure would suggest. Expenditure data also gives no indication of quality or quantity of goods consumed both of which are relevant to any measure of standard of living. The GHS will supplement the FES to create a broader measure by addition of information on, for example, leisure, housing, health.

THE DATA

The FES is an annual survey resulting in a sample of about 7,000 households. There are three main categories of information: personal and demographic; income; expenditure on housing and fuel at a household level; and on other items by means of an individual two-week expenditure diary.

The GHS is also an annual survey resulting in a larger sample size of 10,000 households. Certain core topics are included every year while other topics are included periodically or on an *ad hoc* basis. The core topics include personal and demographic data and in recent years income data similar to that collected in the FES has also been gathered. Core topics can be divided into five main subject areas: family information, housing, education, employment, and health. An occasional topic is leisure activities which was most recently included in 1983. As the FES and the GHS sample different families it is obviously not possible to combine them directly. It is, however, possible to combine them at an aggregate level, that is to match groups of households with similar compositions and income levels in the two data sets and to draw on both for information on their living standards.

USING THE FES AND GHS TO MEASURE STANDARDS OF LIVING

Under Townsend's headings what indicators of standards of living are available in the FES and GHS? Table 12.1 compares Townsend's ideas for an index with information in the FES and GHS.

Between them, the FES and GHS supply information under nearly every head of Townsend's scheme. The major gaps are under the environment and location heads. There are problems with the information available under some other heads also. Expenditure on fuel, for example, only tells us that a certain amount of money is spent on fuel, it does not tell us how warm and comfortable a home is or even how much heat is purchased. This exemplifies Atkinson's problem of unobservable variables. Some information in the FES/GHS bears on the necessities defined in the Mack and Lansley survey, but rather indirectly. For example, direct information is not available on possession of a warm overcoat or on how warm a living area is but likelihood of purchase and amount spent on clothing and fuel is available. Thus on the scope of the indicators available, the information in the FES/GHS falls short of this ideal and what would be included in a specially designed survey.

Other desirable and pragmatic criteria for a measure of standards of living were mentioned by Townsend and other authors who have been concerned with the conceptual issues. These include that: the measures should be objective; the information to construct the index should be available; the measure should be appropriate to the political context of its use; the normative elements should be made clear; the role of the unit of measurement should be made clear; the measure should be applicable to every member of society and ideally across societies; and the duration of different standards of living should be measurable.

184

Table 12.1 Information on standards of living in FES/GHS

TOWNSEND	FES	GHS
(a) *Material deprivation*		
Dietary	Amounts and proportions of expenditure on different foods	
Clothing	Amounts and proportions of expenditure on clothing	
Housing	Expenditure Tenure Rateable value Type of dwelling, size	Amenities Overcrowding Housing satisfaction Whether wants to move
Environment	Little information	
Location	Little information	
(b) *Social deprivation* Rights to employment	Current employment status	Time in that status, job and pay satisfaction, pension rights, overtime and short working hours
Family activities		Visits to friends and relations
Integration in community		Could be inferred from leisure activities such as sports, social clubs, and so on
Formal participation in social institutions		Could be inferred from leisure activities, going to church, voluntary activities
Recreation		Leisure activities: at home (TV, radio, reading, music, sewing, DIY, gardening), going out for meals, drink, sports activities, evening classes
Education		Levels of education achieved Numbers in household participating in education

On some of these qualities of a measure of standard of living, the FES and GHS score well: the questions are mainly objective. Only a few items describe feelings – such as satisfaction with job, pay, and accommodation and these could be omitted if appropriate. The fact that neither is designed to elicit information to construct a deprivation index suggests that the information may describe behaviour with less bias than specially designed surveys.

An index based on the FES/GHS is clearly operational. These data sets are available and repeated every year so that Townsend's concern that the measurement of poverty being specific to a particular time in a given society can be overcome by reworking it when necessary. This way the effect of duration of different standards of living for aggregate groups of households could be inferred although this would not be possible for individual households.

It is not clear at this stage how possible it will be to develop a measure of standard of living which is applicable to every member of society. This might mean developing a blunter instrument than one designed to consider family types separately. It seems likely that the indicators in the FES and GHS, as well as varying with income, will also vary with family type. For example, couples with young children might be more likely to spend their leisure time in the home than childless couples, and young people are likely to have more active leisure pursuits than the elderly. It may be useful, as the analysis progresses, to consider the indicators of living standards at two levels. The first level would consist of indicators that are common to all family types and might include various measures of housing adequacy, access to certain consumer durables, health, certain leisure activities such as visiting friends. The second level would consist of indicators which are specific to a given family type. The advantage of trying to conceptualize the living standard indicators at these two levels (common and specific) is that it might provide a more rigorous way of controlling for taste or preference.

The political context for which this measure is being developed is to provide information about the adequacy of the standard of living allowed by the supplementary benefit system and to do this some knowledge is required of the standard of living in the rest of society to which that of those on SB should relate. The standard of living allowed on SB is the subject of another paper.

UNIT OF ANALYSIS

We have followed the often used practice of considering families as tax units because these are the units to which income and benefit apply. To be clear about shared goods such as housing and heating, single tax unit families have mostly been defined.

Two points should be made at this stage about the unit of analysis. First, both surveys are household surveys and collect no information about the distribution of resources in the households, so although a 'household' may be considered to have a satisfactory standard of living, it has been shown that certain household members, such as women, can be deprived within these households. Second because they are household surveys, non-householders are excluded, hence homeless people, who would without question be included among the poor, are excluded from the study. Also, those in any form of residential care are excluded.

LINKING THE FES AND GHS

The family types chosen for linking the FES and GHS data are derived and developed from the study by O'Higgins *et al.* of income distribution over the life cycle (O'Higgins, Bradshaw, and Walker 1988). In using groups throughout the life cycle we follow a long tradition of the use of the notion of the life cycle in studies of living standards and poverty. All groups have sufficient cases to allow examination of the effects of income on standard of living for a particular type of family. In some cases the numbers in the survey of the particular family type allow division into 10 subgroups based on deciles of the income distribution and in others only into 5 groups based on quintiles. The whole project will study the living standards of family types throughout the life cycle ranging from households of one person aged under 35, through to young couples without children, families of increasing size and age, older couples after the children have left home, to one- and two-person pensioner households. In this paper however, we illustrate with one family type only – one person aged under 35.

EXAMPLES OF LIVING STANDARD INDICATORS FROM
THE FES AND GHS

In this section, the information available in the FES and GHS is used to describe the living standards of a chosen family type at different income levels. The family type used for illustration is single persons aged under 35. This group is chosen because all indicators are relevant and, although in the past it has not been a group of particular concern in a policy context, with the advent of income support, deregulation of rented housing, and high unemployment, the circumstances of this group may be of interest to policy makers. To date similar analyses have been carried out for two other family types: families with all children under 5; and lone elderly women under 80. For brevity, the results of these analyses are only summarized in the final discussion. The indicators investigated here concern detailed expenditure on diet, expenditure on the main commodities, some individual items of expenditure from the FES, followed by indicators from the GHS on employment, housing, leisure, and health. In considering the indicators, we are looking for those that vary substantially over the income distribution and for any which give evidence of a threshold.

Diet

Information is gathered on a much more comprehensive list of food items in the FES than has been analysed so far, and this will be analysed in due course. Some trends emerge from the sub-set of food items analysed at this stage: those with lower incomes are more likely to buy eggs, margarine, milk; whereas those with higher incomes are more likely to consume butter, cheese, and possibly fresh fruit. The amounts spent on fresh fruit and vegetables by the higher income groups are greater.

Other expenditure items

Table 12.2 shows the proportions and amounts spent at different income levels on the main commodity heads in the FES. Higher income households are more likely to have spent something in the diary fortnight on every commodity except tobacco and possibly alcohol. It could be inferred from this that higher income, not unex-

Table 12.2   Single person age under 35: expenditure on main commodities,
£ per week (FES)

| | Quintiles | | | | |
	1	2	3	4	5
Fuel	4.56 (92)*	4.57 (86)	6.01 (94)	5.18 (92)	6.76 (96)
Food	10.13 (100)	13.83 (100)	15.17 (100)	16.26 (100)	16.74 (100)
Alcohol	5.60 (72)	5.93 (84)	7.91 (92)	10.86 (84)	10.32 (90)
Tobacco	4.13 (58)	4.31 (36)	5.78 (34)	4.83 (34)	7.05 (26)
Clothing and footwear	9.79 (34)	10.57 (50)	8.38 (52)	12.83 (58)	21.99 (50)
Durable h/h goods	2.43 (50)	6.68 (64)	4.63 (80)	9.16 (86)	25.39 (92)
Other goods	4.49 (100)	4.47 (100)	4.75 (100)	8.46 (98)	11.82 (100)
Transport	5.02 (54)	7.75 (84)	13.43 (100)	17.76 (94)	22.77 (96)
Services	3.59 (84)	6.28 (100)	7.93 (100)	18.60 (100)	20.38 (100)

* Figures in brackets are proportion puchasing

pectedly, increases choice. Clearly the greater likelihood of expenditure on tobacco causes problems for including this as a behavioural indicator of poverty, and recalls questions asked earlier – if low income households can afford to spend on tobacco can they be said not to be able to afford to spend enough on food? Even though the proportion buying any commodity may or may not increase with income, the amount spent certainly does and for every commodity, although the range of expenditure is more variable for some commodities than others.

Rights to employment

Over three-quarters of those in the lowest quintile were out of work compared with a few cases in the rest of the distribution. Only one person in the lowest quintile was a member of an occupational pension scheme but the proportion rose rapidly to 86 per cent in the fourth and fifth quintiles. A similar pattern is observed with satisfaction with the job although the highest percentage (76 per cent) of those saying they were satisfied was reached by those in the third quintile. Satisfaction with pay increased entirely predictably with increase in income but only in the top quintile were more than two-thirds satisfied with pay.

Housing and amenities (Table 12.3)

Clearly the extent of owner-occupation varies with income for this family type. The indicator chosen for the type of housing does not illustrate very definitely where people are living except that as income rises fewer households live in flats. Ownership of a telephone and a car increase steadily with income but the ownership of gas central heating seems to alter more discretely with income.

Health (Table 12.4)

It can be said that, in general, those with higher incomes enjoy better health and vice versa. Those in the lowest quintile do seem to be considerably more likely to suffer a long-standing illness than those in the rest of the income distribution. This is one of the few indicators we have looked at so far for which the threshold hypothesis might hold.

Leisure activities (Table 12.5)

The leisure activities which varied most noticeably with income were going out for a meal or a drink, and the proportion reading books as an activity rose substantially from the first to second quintile.

Higher income people were less likely to undertake no activities and the debate about choice and taste may be highlighted by the other commonly mentioned activities in that billiards features more often in the lower quintiles and squash, athletics, and swimming are more often mentioned by the higher income groups.

Grouped Indicators (Figure 12.1, Table 12.6)

Figure 12.1 shows how a group of indicators, each of which varies individually with income, vary jointly: health, having a telephone, car ownership, going out for a meal; and having a job. The lack of a job seems to be the only indicator consistent with the threshold idea.

An alternative approach is to describe what the living standard of people at different income levels includes or allows, and Table 12.6 attempts this. Overlaps are clear but distinguishing features also emerge.

Table 12.3   Single person under 35: housing and amenities (FES)

	Quintiles				
	1	2	3	4	5
					percentages
In owner					
occupation	4 cases	2 cases	35	60	84
Living in:					
(i) semi	2 cases	6 cases	9 cases	8 cases	5 cases
(ii) flat	78	72	59	58	50
(iii) terraced	4 cases	8 cases	22	8 cases	30
Proportion with:					
telephone	20	48	53	82	86
car	20	20	45	58	66
gas CH	32	40	41	42	58
fridge/freezer	62	76	69	74	66
freezer	5 cases	4 cases	5 cases	5 cases	8 cases

Table 12.4   Single person under 35: health (GHS)

	Quintiles				
	1	2	3	4	5
					percentages
General health					
good	61	70	66	80	80
not good	3 cases	4 cases	4 cases	2 cases	None
Long-standing					
illness	37	30	32	28	27
Had to cut down					
activities in					
past fortnight					
because of					
illness	8 cases	6 cases	4 cases	7 cases	2 cases

SUMMARY AND CONCLUDING REMARKS

Townsend's ideas and the subsequent debate on measuring poverty have been reviewed. In the light of this review the possibilities and constraints of using the indicators available in the FES and GHS for a measure of living standards have been considered. Information on most indicators proposed in the literature is available in one form or another in the FES/GHS. The major gaps are information on the environment and location. The information available in the FES/GHS also meets other criteria for the development of a measure of standards of living such as objectivity and availability.

The possibility of using these data is illustrated for one family type,

Table 12.5 Leisure activities for a single person under 35 (GHS)

	Quintiles				
	1	*2*	*3*	*4*	*5*
					percentages
Watched TV	96	96	100	96	96
Listened to radio	86	92	90	96	96
Listened to records	86	88	90	88	92
Read books	51	74	74	80	76
Visited friends or were visited	92	92	96	98	98
Out for meal (not in working hours)	45	62	74	76	82
Out for drink (not in working hours)	78	94	96	88	94
Gardening	33	22	30	32	39
Sewing	9 cases	32	18	12	16
DIY	47	30	62	62	51

Number of activities

| | Cases | | | | |
none	6 cases	6 cases	9 cases	3 cases	4 cases
1	8	9	4	6	3
2	9	7	8	12	6
3	6	7	6	9	9
4	5	10	6	5	9
5	9	9	6	4	6
6+	6	2	11	11	12

Most common
1st activity:

6 cases	6 cases	9 cases	3 cases	4 cases
o/walk 10	o/walk 15	o/walk 5	camp. caravan 5	o/walk 11
billrds 6	badmin. 3	athltcs 3	soccer 5	athltcs 3
		billrds 3		squash 3
				swim. 3

2nd activity:

6 cases	6 cases	9 cases	3 cases	4 cases
o/walk 5	squash 5	films 4	dancing 4	swim. 6
billrds 4	swim. 4	swim. 3	films 4	o/walk 4
		billrds 3		squash 4
		darts 3		hobbies 4

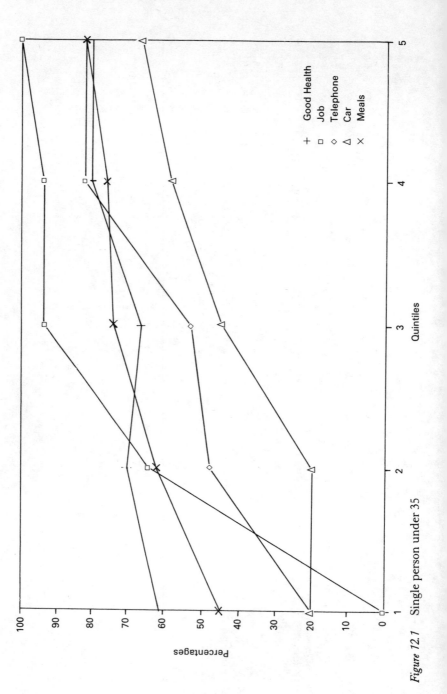

Figure 12.1 Single person under 35

Legend:
+ Good Health
□ Job
◇ Telephone
△ Car
× Meals

Percentages

Quintiles

Table 12.6   Single people under 35: standards of living at different income levels

	No job 100%	Good health 60%	Telephone 20%	Gas CH 32%
LOWEST QUINTILE	Commodities: more likely to spend on: tobacco			
	Diet: more likely to include: margarine, eggs, cooked meat			
	Leisure: read books 51%, out for meal 45%, drink 78%			
	Car 20%	Flat 70%		

	No job 66%	Good health 70%	Telephone 48%	Gas CH 40%
NEXT QUINTILE	Commodities: more likely to spend on: alcohol, durables, transport, clothes			
	spends more on clothing, durables, transport			
	Diet: more likely to include: beef, frozen fish, butter, cheese, fresh vegetables, fruit			
	Leisure: read books 75%, out for drink 94%, sewing 32%			

	Job 100%	Good health 80%	Telephone 86%	Gas CH 58%
HIGHEST QUINTILE	Commodities: spends even more on clothing, durables, transport			
	Leisure: out for meal 82%			
	Car 66%	Flat 50%		

single persons under 35, and indicators such as expenditure on various commodities, whether working, leisure, or health are investigated for variation over income and evidence of a threshold. Of the indicators investigated so far, the one that varies most strikingly with income is whether working or not. This raises the question of cause and effect, and the status of such an indicator *vis à vis* the others discussed. Townsend includes employment rights in his poverty index and lack of work is clearly a major form of exclusion from society, but future research will need to discuss how valid it is to include it in an index which is then correlated with income.

Other indicators which clearly vary with income are owner-occupation, having a telephone and a car. Higher income households spend more on all commodities and are more likely to purchase any commodity except tobacco. Some evidence of difference in diet at different income levels was also demonstrated. Of the subjective indicators, health and satisfaction with work both varied with income.

It is worth mentioning briefly the results from the similar exercise carried out on two additional family types: families with all children under 5 and lone elderly women under 80. Some indicators did seem to be common to all three family types: the greater amounts spent on all commodity items, the greater use of domestic service and owner occupation as income rose. As anticipated, some indicators did seem to be specific to particular groups. Health and employment rights were specific to single people under 35 and the husbands in the families with children under 5. Among leisure activities indicators specific to particular family types were: going out for a meal for people under 35, listening to the radio or records or reading for husbands and wives in families with children under five.

Evidence of a threshold seems to exist for some indicators at various points on the income scale for each indicator. It is not clear at this stage, however, how many of these indicators would coalesce to form a clear pattern of a threshold at one level of income which could then be designated as the 'poverty line'. An impression of the data suggests that the pattern is rather like that described by Okun:

> A short trip from the dreary slums to the classy areas of the suburbs is an interplanetary voyage measured in economic differentials. But it takes the traveller through a lot of territory occupied by the middle class, whose economic status is neither dreary nor classy.

(Okun 1980)

It seems that on some indicators there is a substantial change from those at the lowest income levels to the middle bands and for others the more noticeable change is from the low and middle bands to the highest income levels. Examples of the first are the employment rights and health indicators and of the second are purchase of fresh fruit and use of domestic services.

More detailed work is required on all expenditure items in the FES, particularly, food items and educational achievements should be included. Eventually we hope to develop an index of living stan-

196

dard using multivariate statistical techniques such as principal components or cluster analysis as Heddy has done on the survey of the unemployed (Heddy 1987).

The conclusion can only take the form of a progress report at this stage. The test of Townsend is under way and the information in the FES and GHS can go some way to developing a measure of living standards. Distilling this information into manageable and comprehensible form requires further work but at least we have improved on Pigou (quoted in Sen 1987) who gave up the objective approach to measure minimum real income because 'it would be necessary to obtain and to analyse a mass of detailed information'.

NOTE

1 The research in this paper was funded by the ESRC. Material from the General Household Survey made available through the office of Population, Census and Surveys and the ESRC Data Archive has been used by permission of the Controller of HM Stationery Office. The author would like to thank Carol Propper for comments.

REFERENCES

Abel-Smith, B. and Townsend, P. (1965) *The Poor and the Poorest*, London: Bell.

Ashton, P. (1984) 'Poverty and its beholders', *New Society* (18 October).

Atkinson, A.B. (1980) *Wealth, Income and Inequality*, Oxford: Oxford University Press.

Atkinson, A. B. (1974) 'Poverty and income, inequality in Britain', in D. Wedderburn (ed.), *Poverty, Inequality and Class Structure*, Cambridge: Cambridge University Press.

Atkinson, A. B. (1984) 'How should we measure poverty?: some conceptual issues', Paper for symposium on the measurement of poverty, Berlin.

Bradshaw, J., Cooke, K., and Godfrey, C. (1984) 'The impact of unemployment on the living standards of families', *Journal of Social Policy* 12 (4).

Bradshaw, J. and Morgan, J. (1987) *Budgetting on Benefit*, London: Family Policy Studies Centre.

Fiegehen, G., Lansley, S., and Smith, A. (1977) *Poverty and Progress in Britain 1953–1973*, Cambridge: Cambridge University Press.

Heddy, P. (1987) Unpublished RSS Paper on measuring living standards in the DHSS/OPCS survey of unemployment and living standards.

Mack, J. and Lansley, S. (1985) *Poor Britain*, London: George Allen & Unwin.

Nicholson, J. (1979) 'The assessment of poverty and the information we need in social security research: the definition and measurement of poverty', DHSS, London: HMSO.

O'Higgins, M., Bradshaw, J., and Walker, R. (1988) 'Income distribution over the life cycle', in R. Walker and G. Parker (eds), *Money Matters*, London: Sage.

Okun, A. M. (1980) 'Equality of income and opportunity', in A. B. Atkinson (ed.) *Wealth, Income and Inequality*, Oxford: Oxford University Press.

Piachaud, D. (1981) 'Peter Townsend and the Holy Grail', *New Society*, (10 September).

Piachaud, D. (1987) 'Problems in the definitions and measurement of poverty', *Journal of Social Policy*, 16 (2):147–64.

Rowntree, B. S. (1901) *Poverty: A Study of Town Life*, London: Macmillan.

Sen, A. (1987) 'The standard of living: lecture 1, concepts and critiques', in G. Hawthorn (ed.) *The Standard of Living*, Cambridge: Cambridge University Press.

Townsend, P. (1979) *Poverty in the United Kingdom*, Harmondsworth: Penguin Books.

Townsend, P. (1987) 'Deprivation', *Journal of Social Policy*, 16, (2):125–46.

Part Four

POLICY ISSUES

THE RELATIONSHIP BETWEEN INDIVIDUAL CHOICE AND GOVERNMENT POLICY IN THE DECISION TO CONSUME HAZARDOUS GOODS

CHRISTINE GODFREY and MELANIE POWELL

INTRODUCTION

Public health has been an important target for government policy throughout the nineteenth and twentieth centuries. Basic improvements in sanitation and the working environment have reduced mortality rates from major causes of deaths such as infectious diseases, and have increased population longevity. The effect of these policies has been to improve quality of life for the majority. Given these basic improvements, more recent public health policy has focused on the link between changing patterns of consumption and the incidence of disease. In particular, tobacco use has been associated with lung cancer and bronchitis, and alcohol use with liver cirrhosis and digestive disorders. It is now claimed that the quality of life should be improved still further by government action to restrict the individual's freedom to consume hazardous goods in order to reduce the levels of associated harm within the population (see, for example, reports from the Royal College of Psychiatrists 1979, 1986; the World Health Organization 1985; the Royal College of Physicians 1983; the Royal College of General Practitioners 1986).

An economic rationale explaining the use of government policy to improve the quality of life by restricting individual choice in the consumption of hazardous goods is examined in this paper using the examples of alcohol and tobacco. The relationship between consumption of these hazardous goods and changes in the quality of life for individual consumers and society in general is examined in

201

section one. A basic economic model of the role of government policy in restricting consumer choice is then outlined and discussed in the second section. The applicability of the economic model for designing and evaluating policies to restrict consumer choice and increase quality of life, however, depends upon the relevance of the basic assumptions of the economic model. The value judgements that underpin these assumptions are therefore examined in relation to alcohol and tobacco use in the final section.

QUALITY OF LIFE AND THE CONSUMPTION OF ALCOHOL AND TOBACCO

From an economic perspective, the quality of life is a measure of the overall level of satisfaction gained from the consumption and production of goods and services. The consumption of alcohol and tobacco confers benefits on consumers by satisfying physical, psychological, and social needs. These benefits raise the individual's valuation of the quality of life and add to general well-being or welfare in society. However, there is always a cost attached to the acquisition of benefits which offsets the total gain. The most obvious cost is the price paid or the sacrifice of some other form of expenditure or saving. Hazardous goods are those which carry additional costs in the form of adverse physical and social consequences. These costs reduce welfare in society by decreasing the individual's valuation of quality of life when the consumer is ill-informed or addicted, and by reducing the quality of life of third parties who may also bear the costs. The problems associated with the identification of the costs of alcohol and tobacco are discussed in this section together with the problems of measuring benefits against which costs must be set.

Measuring the harm

The results of multidisciplinary research into the harmful consequences of alcohol and tobacco consumption have led to the identification of three types of harm as presented in Figure 13.1. Medical factors are particularly prominent, comprising estimates of the morbidity and mortality resulting from alcohol and tobacco use. However, there are also important non-health consequences which have been classified as social and legal problems (Thorley 1982).

202

Figure 13.1 Examples of the harmful consequences of alcohol and tobacco consumption

Type of harm	Associated consumption pattern	ALCOHOL		TOBACCO	
		Individual effect	Third party effect	Individual effect	Third party effect
Medical	Acute	Intoxication/ poisoning	Emergency care	Coughing/ dizzyness	
	Continued	Cirrhosis/ Brain damage	Caring for disabled	Bronchitis/ Sinusitis	Passive smoking
	Chronic	Alcohol dependence syndrome	Death of drinker	Lung cancer/ heart disease	Death of smoker
Social	Acute	Loss of belongings	Domestic violence	Derision/loss of face	Concern
	Continued	Financial debt	Sexual Problems	Smelling unpleasant	Irritation
	Chronic	Stigma	Marital breakdown	Inability to function without a cigarette	Fire hazards
Legal	Acute	Charged for criminal offence	Victim of assault	Underaged consumption	Sale of tobacco to minor
	Continued	Removal of licence for drunk driving	Road traffic accident	Avoidance of non-smoking areas	Designation of property rights
	Chronic	Vagrancy/ forced withdrawal	Public order	Compensation suits	Compensation payments

The two other characteristics of harm are that costs may fall on the individual consumer or on third parties, and that costs may occur concurrently with consumption or be related to past consumption patterns. Measurement of many of these problems, particularly intangible factors such as the pain, grief, and suffering attached to any premature death, is extremely difficult.

Estimates of the number of deaths associated with alcohol, tobacco, and illicit drugs are widely used as indicators of the adverse effects of consumption. Figures in Table 13.1 show tobacco-related deaths to be a major cause of premature mortality, with 63 per cent of the total number of deaths being attributed to lung cancer and 36 per cent to coronary heart disease. Differences between estimates of alcohol-related deaths reflect the variety of diseases with which alcohol is related and the paucity of epidemiological studies (see McDonnell and Maynard 1985a).

The alcohol mortality rates shown in Table 13.1, unlike those for drugs and tobacco, include the deaths of third parties which result from individual drinking behaviour. An example would be the deaths of passengers and other victims resulting from a drink-related road traffic accident. Some indirect third party deaths, however, could also be associated with smoking. It has been estimated that lung cancers arising from passive smoking, for example, may be of the order of 200 cases per year (Green College Consensus 1987) and that smoking and alcohol are separate and joint contributory factors in accidental fires (Tether and Harrison 1986) and road accidents (Waller 1986).

Mortality figures indicate the rate of premature deaths occurring in any given period. Perhaps a more appropriate indicator of the costs to health of consumption would be a measure of potential life years lost (see McDonnell and Maynard 1985b). However, life years lost as a measure of costs are not adjusted for quality of life, thereby failing to measure the impact of other costs identified in Figure 13.1.

Table 13.1   Estimates of mortality

	Estimated Number of deaths	Source of Data	Year of data
Illicit drugs	127	DHSS (1985)	1982
	235	BMJ (1986)	1984
Alcohol	5,013–7,887	McDonnell and Maynard (1985b)	1983
	25,000	BMJ (1986)	1984
	4,000	Royal College of Psychiatrists (1986)	1983
	40,000	Royal College of General Practitioners (1986)	1984
	25,000	Royal College of Physicians (1987)	NK
Tobacco	100,000	Royal College of Physicians (1983)	1981

Source: Maynard, Hardman, and Whelan (1987).

Many types of associated harm, including mortality, show a strong correlation over time with consumption. Per capita consumption has therefore been used as an indicator for general cost levels across the population. For alcohol, this has been formalized using a statistical relationship (Ledermann 1956). Although per capita figures may indicate trends in costs, there is no obvious relationship between consumption and the value of costs at any time.

Several attempts have therefore been made in economic studies to estimate the monetary value of the annual total costs to society. Some typical results for alcohol are shown in Table 13.2. The total estimate includes the value of costs which result directly from alcohol consumption such as resources used in health care, and also the value of costs which are indirectly associated with consumption such as lost output. Detailed studies of smoking are not available for the UK although the Government estimates that the cost to the NHS of smoking-related illness was of the order of £209m to £500m in 1985-6 (Maynard, Hardman, and Whelan 1987).

The interpretation of total cost figures is open to question (Godfrey and Powell 1987). For example, no distinction is made between those who bear the burden of costs in an estimate of total cost. The cost of reduced productivity caused by smoking or alcohol in the form of sickness absence, absenteeism, or lower productivity at work may be partly experienced by the individual in the form of lower earnings, partly by the employers through lower profits, or by other workers through lower wages. Similarly, part of the cost of alcohol-related traffic accidents is reflected in insurance premiums

Table 13.2 The resource costs of alcohol misuse, England and Wales (1985 prices)

		£m
Social cost to industry – Total		1592.20
Sickness absence		(723.55)
Premature deaths		(166.74)
Unemployment		(653.31)
Social costs to the National Health Service		112.12
Society's response to alcohol-related problems		0.93
Social cost of material damage		104.01
Social costs of criminal activities		37.57
	Total	1846.83

Source: Maynard, Hardman, and Whelan (1987).

205

levied on non-drinking drivers. These effects are in addition to the direct harm caused to third parties by passive smoking, irritation and nuisance, and from drink-driving and public disturbances. The costing figures presented in Table 13.1 are derived from one type of costing methodology used in public health analysis. Many studies have adopted alternative approaches, but face similar problems (Godfrey and Powell 1987). Total costs can be viewed as an index of potential reductions in the quality of life, weighted by their market valuation, but the index is often incomplete or based on arbitrary assumptions and must therefore be treated with caution.

Measuring the benefits

The benefits of alcohol and tobacco consumption are an index of potential improvements in the quality of life of the consumer. There may also be benefits for those in contact with consumers, for example, the role of alcohol in social communication. As benefits take the form of psycho-social effects, they are difficult to quantify. The impact of these benefits on the quality of life may be valued using expenditure data, as expenditure represents the consumers' valuation or willingness to pay for the benefits. As some individuals are willing to pay a higher price than the current level, expenditure measures may understate the value of benefits from consumption. If consumers are unaware of the risks from consuming hazardous goods, however, or are addicted or dependent, then expenditure may overstate the value of benefits.

The real value of tobacco expenditure and the share of tobacco expenditure in total consumer expenditure has fallen substantially since 1973, both as a real value and as a share in total consumer expenditure. By comparison real expenditure on alcohol grew steadily from 1960 to 1979, declined during the economic recession, but began to recover after 1982. Consumer expenditure on alcohol was £16,474m in 1986 and comprised 7 per cent of total consumer expenditure, with more money being spent on alcohol than on clothing and foot-wear (see Central Statistical Office 1987). Consumer expenditure on tobacco was £7,471m in 1986, 3.2 per cent of total consumer expenditure.

The distribution of costs and benefits

The data presented above are insufficient to establish either the

206

distribution of costs and benefits or to identify those individuals whose quality of life is directly affected by the consumption of alcohol and tobacco. In this section some of the available evidence is considered. In 1961 a survey by the Tobacco Advisory Council (TAC) suggested that 72 per cent of men smoked. Surveys indicate that there has been a considerable decline in the number of individuals who smoke and by 1984 smokers formed a minority in all gender and social classes (General Household Survey 1986).

The decline in smoking was not uniform and, particularly for men, there were large social class differences in smoking behaviour by 1984 (GHS 1986). The health effects of the current distribution of consumption, after a time, will be reflected in future mortality statistics. In addition, the results of the recent *Health and Lifestyle Survey* (1987) show links between current smoking and current malaise and illness measures.

Surveys of drinking behaviour suggest that the majority of people drink, if only occasionally. The Wilson (1980) survey suggested that 6 per cent of men and 11 per cent of women in England and Wales were non-drinkers. Additionally, about 18 per cent of men and 31 per cent of women were occasional or infrequent drinkers. Similar figures were obtained in the GHS survey for that year, and more recent GHS data suggest there have been few substantial changes in male drinking habits. Dunbar and Morgan (1987), however, suggest that although the number of women drinkers in England and Wales has fallen since 1978, the average alcohol consumption per woman drinker in 1985 was significantly higher. These figures may indicate a future rise in the number of alcohol-related diseases among women as women are susceptible to alcohol-related damage at lower consumption levels than men.

Data from the 1985 Family Expenditure Survey (FES) are presented in Table 13.3 as an illustration of how smoking and drinking, jointly and separately, may influence the quality of life of households as well as individuals. Participation rates vary between households as well as individuals. Figures in Table 13.3 illustrate the differences between households headed by a retired person and all other households. The figures for average expenditure and the share of alcohol and tobacco expenditure in the total budget outline the variations in patterns of expenditure between households with different consumption habits. So, for example, for 'smoking and drinking' non-retired headed households, the combined expendi-

Table 13.3   Household expenditure on alcohol and tobacco, 1985

Household type classified by expenditure pattern	Households headed by a retired person		Households headed by a non-retired person	
A. Number of households of different types	Number	%	Number	%
No alcohol or tobacco expenditure	489	41.4	692	12.7
Both alcohol and tobacco expenditure	385	24.6	2400	44.1
Tobacco expenditure but no alcohol expenditure	229	14.6	504	9.3
Alcohol expenditure but no tobacco expenditure	463	29.6	1850	34.0
B. Average alcohol expenditure	£ per week		£ per week	
Both alcohol and tobacco expenditure	8.68		13.56	
Alcohol expenditure but no tobacco expenditure	5.89		9.25	
C. Average tobacco expenditure	£ per week		£ per week	
Both alcohol and tobacco expenditure	7.10		9.63	
Tobacco expenditure but no alcohol expenditure	4.87		8.04	
D. Alcohol expenditure as a proportion of total expenditure	%		%	
Both alcohol and tobacco expenditure	7.8		7.6	
Alcohol expenditure but no tobacco expenditure	6.5		5.5	
E. Tobacco expenditure as a proportion of total expenditure	%		%	
Both alcohol and tobacco expenditure	7.6		6.5	
Tobacco expenditure but no alcohol expenditure	8.0		9.4	
Total number of households in group	1566		5446	

Source: Family Expenditure Survey Data (1985).

ture on alcohol and tobacco accounts on average for over 14 per cent of the total weekly household expenditure. For retired headed households the proportion is even larger with an average of over 15 per cent of total household expenditure being spent on these products. Further analyses of FES data show there are more smokers and smokers and drinkers in lower income groups over a wide range of household types. Smoking and drinking behaviour can therefore have a major impact on families' budgets, particularly for those households which contain one or more persons who are both heavy drinkers and smokers.

ECONOMIC MODEL OF WELFARE, CONSUMER CHOICE AND GOVERNMENT INTERVENTION

From the economic perspective, the quality of life is an element of individual welfare which can be improved through market trade and consumption. If every individual is capable of judging how best to improve their quality of life and welfare, unrestricted trade in all goods including hazardous goods, can lead to (one definition of) a maximum level of welfare. This abstract model is used as a 'benchmark' against which to compare real world market behaviour by individuals. When the two diverge, government intervention may be warranted. Government policy aimed at restricting consumer choice, therefore, involves a collective decision to override the sovereignty of individual choice to determine quality of life.

In this section, the underlying assumptions of the economic benchmark model are discussed together with the 'market failure' explanations for intervention in alcohol and tobacco markets. Given the underlying assumptions of the economic model, a theoretical link between individual choice and government restrictions is developed. The resulting framework provides a basis for comparing different policies by measuring changes in costs and benefits to individuals and the overall impact on social welfare.

The economic model

A criticism frequently lodged against the economic model is that it does not realistically describe individual behaviour. However, a model need be neither realistic nor universal, but should provide a simplified version of reality which aids understanding and prediction of behaviour. The economic model relates to individual choice and is based on two fundamental behavioural assumptions which describe the consumer's rationality and sovereignty. (Varian 1978:ch.3).

209

Rationality does not involve any notion of 'normal' behaviour in a given set of circumstances. It means that consumers do and can choose to maximize their own welfare with full information. Welfare is the net benefit derived by individuals from their consumption; the benefits of choice net of the costs of making that choice. Rationality ensures that individuals consume goods to improve their overall level of welfare, so that they consume all goods up to the point where additional benefits just balance the additional costs.

The economic benchmark model is one in which individuals can trade freely, given the behavioural assumptions, up to the limits of their income. Trade takes place in markets which work perfectly, in which no individual can exert monopoly power, in which no individual's choice will result in others involuntarily bearing the cost, and in which everyone has all the information required to make a choice. If an economy functioned in this way, it would result in an efficient allocation of goods and services between individuals. Efficiency implies that there is no alternative allocation which would improve the welfare of any individual without reducing the welfare of someone else. Because the economic model incorporates rationality and consumer sovereignty, no third party is needed to determine when or if someone is better or worse off. Social welfare is determined by individuals through trade. It is only when markets fail to function perfectly that social welfare and individual welfare can be improved by government intervention.

The market failure model

Market failures can be categorized into two types: monopoly power where consumers or producers can distort prices which would otherwise be set by market forces; and externalities (and public goods) where individual choice results in benefits or costs to third parties which are not traded. Examples of both kinds of market failure can be identified in the alcohol and tobacco markets, forming the basis of the economic rationale which can be used to explain the need for intervention in the choice to consume these goods.

A few large companies dominate production of both alcohol and tobacco. Economic theory predicts that these companies may compete on the basis of non-price competition, for example by advertising. Extreme levels of advertising may increase overall demand or project false or biased information. As a result, consumption of alcohol and tobacco may be too high relative to the level associated with the benchmark model. In addition producers may not wish to disseminate information about the long-run health effects of alcohol and tobacco. Government may therefore choose to control aspects of the supply of these goods such as advertising, health information, and producer market concentration.

The market for information in the real world is far from perfect, particularly in relation to the uncertainty and risks involved in the consumption of alcohol and tobacco. One important factor results from the long time-period which may elapse between consumption and manifestations of harmful consequences. These imperfections when combined with failure in the health care market, for example, may lead to distorted consumer choice. Government could choose to improve information on the private costs of consumption to the individual, provide health care, or improve private market provision of both.

One of the most frequently cited justifications for government control over individual choice to consume alcohol or tobacco is the existence of external costs to third parties. If external costs arise from passive smoking and harm to innocent victims of a drunk driver, for example, individuals will calculate a higher rate of net benefits from drinking and smoking than the actual social rate. As a result, they will consume more tobacco and alcohol than the efficient level. The policy response may be to levy a tax, or impose regulations to limit consumption. Licence restrictions on the sale of alcohol might be interpreted in this way.

The market failure model can be used to identify both a reason for government intervention and the most appropriate policy target. However, some positive level of harm from the consumption of hazardous goods might exist in the efficient solution. The goal of efficiency is to balance the costs and benefits at the margin of choice rather than to eliminate all costs.

Efficiency, equity, and value judgements

Efficiency is the objective derived from the economic model, but, in a complex, imperfect market, absolute efficiency cannot be practically identified or achieved. The policy criteria for hazardous goods must therefore be commuted to relative efficiency through the identification of an improvement in welfare. In the study of welfare economics, a framework has been developed in which one state of the world can be deemed 'better' than another. Comparisons between alcohol and tobacco policies, for example, could be made by calculating social welfare as an aggregate function of individual preferences in alternative states using cost-benefit techniques. Measures of costs and benefits such as those discussed in section one would be used. However, evaluation is dependent upon the criteria used. In general, if those who gain from a change in alcohol policy could more than compensate the losers, social welfare is said to rise and the policy involves an efficient move. This criterion involves additional assumptions.

Equity considerations relate to the distribution of gains and losses between people arising from a policy change. Changes in equity cannot be evaluated without further assumptions to attach differential weights to individual gainers or losers. Alcohol and tobacco policy is 'loaded' with equity issues about property rights to 'clean air', about liberty and freedom to choose, and about the moral value of alcohol in society. The predictive and evaluative power of economic analysis of policy change are unclear unless the additional equity assumptions are made explicit.

THE RELEVANCE OF THE ECONOMIC MODEL IN POLICY ISSUES RELATING TO HAZARDOUS GOODS

The economic model outlined in the previous section utilized two types of value judgements: assumptions about the behaviour of individuals and assumptions about the nature of the market for trade. In the case where the hazard in consumption is potentially addictive it could be argued that these assumptions are not relevant. If the basic assumptions do not provide a functional model with predictive power, the economic model can offer little insight into policy decisions. It is argued here that the basic model can be extended and the assumptions relaxed in order to accommodate consumption of hazardous goods.

Behavioural assumptions

A simple criticism of the basic economic model would be that the behavioural assumptions which comprise consumer 'rationality' cannot hold when the consumer is addicted. If an individual continues to drink alcohol knowing that more consumption can only lead to a deterioration in their mental and physical well-being the individual cannot be acting rationally. This definition of addiction implies that there are no benefits to be gained from drinking when addicted. The net benefit of consumption, given a positive level of costs, must always be negative and individual welfare will be reduced by further consumption. Addiction therefore involves irrational consumption decisions.

In general, it is accepted that some members of society are not capable of making rational economic decisions, for example, children and adults suffering from mental illness. Paternalist policies involve government acting collectively to override the individual's choice and to define the individual's best interest. In the case of addiction, this could result in a policy to enforce withdrawal and limit future access to the hazardous good. It is not clear, however, that a universal definition of addiction exists. In fact the term addiction has been dropped from the International Classification of Diseases in favour of a general syndrome of dependence (*International Classification of Diseases* 1979). The definition of addiction has changed with the moral climate of society from a weakness of will and sin to physical disease and more recently to social factors in consumption.

However, if consumer choice is modelled as dynamic choice over time, the problem of the relevance of behavioural assumptions in the economic model can be overcome. Dependence could result from rational consumption over time when individuals choose to place a high weight on the benefits of current consumption (avoidance of withdrawal costs, etc.) and a low weight on future costs (health and social problems). Consumers continuously attempt to delay experiencing costs which fall a long period after consumption. In such circumstances individuals may 'demand' policies such as taxation to help them make difficult choices. This has been demonstrated theoretically to be a 'rational choice' by Crain, Deaton, Holcombe, and Tollison (1977) and also can be observed in smokers' attitudes to tobacco taxation (see Leedham 1987).

The economic model can be further extended to overcome the problem of addiction and rationality, by the relaxation of the assumption of full information. Individual choices can be rational over time providing the aim is to maximize the expected level of benefit given all the existing information available at the time of decision making. The health impact of smoking, for example, may be valued at a low level by the very young who have limited information and experience. However, the very old may also place a low value on health despite knowledge and experience because the health effects have limited importance with a short life expectancy (see Wright 1987). Smoking and drinking patterns would therefore be expected to vary over the lifetime of any individual.

Market assumptions

The efficiency criterion is derived from the assumption that individuals will engage in voluntary market exchange to raise their own level of welfare. Market assumptions about consumer sovereignty and the superiority of market allocation mechanisms result from the individualistic approach adopted in the economic model. Society and social welfare are modelled as aggregate functions of individual actions. The individual's freedom to choose is therefore fundamentally important. All the policy prescriptions which arise from the economic models involve actions by government to promote or to constrain individual activity to the efficient level that would obtain in a free market. The desirability of efficiency and government policy to achieve that end depends upon the desirability of the initial value judgements of free trade.

Littlechild and Wiseman (1986) argue that the value judgements about market behaviour may not be directly relevant to policies aimed at restricting individual choice. The economic model takes social values and initial purchasing power as given and cannot be used to analyse questions about who should have rights. These questions involve distributional judgements which are not incorporated in the economic model. In the case of alcohol and tobacco consumption, the allocation of rights depends on current morality and social attitudes. These may support individual rights or define individual choice as 'wrong' (rather than inefficient) for some goods.

Two alternative frameworks for analysing government policies to restrict consumer choice were identified by Littlechild and Wiseman (1986). Paternalism allows government to impose an accepted social valuation of the net benefits of consumption on any individual, while liberalism allows government no freedom to restrict choice except when agreed by all. Depending on the policy issue, these frameworks may lead to conflicting or complementary policy implications. For this reason, Littlechild and Wiseman suggest a public choice approach where the economic model is applied to the analysis of the acceptability of the process from which policies arise rather than the evaluation of policy outcome. The public choice approach examines the process by which governments reach decisions on policy. Institutional decisions are modelled as if they were market transactions. The aim is to model how individual values become enshrined as social values implied by government actions. This is an important but underdeveloped area of economic analysis for the case of alcohol and tobacco.

CONCLUSION

Any analysis of government policy on alcohol and tobacco consumption will involve normative issues of evaluation and the distribution of rights and power amongst individuals. The economic model of market failure takes the existing distribution of power, rights, incomes, and institutions as given. It can be used to investigate 'positive' empirical questions about distributional effects of policy or to evaluate the outcome of any policy in terms of relative efficiency.

Individuals all place different values on costs and benefits of drinking and smoking. Some may be libertarian and place a higher value on the benefits of the right to choose, others may place a low value on the right to choose and prefer a smoke- and drink-free world. Paternalist or libertarian values can be included within the economic model in so far as these factors determine the weights individuals place on the costs and benefits of consumption. From a public choice perspective, as the majority values shift, the nature of the efficient allocation will also change.

The values or moral attitudes that individuals hold about smoking and drinking behaviour also affect the policy implications of the market failure model. For example, the model predicts that government intervention is justified in the presence of externalities, providing the costs of intervention do not outweigh the benefits gained. The value of the externality, however, will be affected by the social values of individuals who make up society. Drunkenness in one society may have more or less impact as an externality than in any other. Different values about equity, rights, and morals alter the shape of the social welfare function that forms the starting point of the market failure model.

An economic approach to the relationship between individual choice in the consumption of hazardous goods and government policy therefore serves several important functions. It can be used to set out a precise definition of social problems and policy responses. The framework also helps analysts to identify and develop new forms of interventions. As a predictive model, economics can be used to investigate positive empirical questions about the consequences of policy change. More importantly, the framework provides a standard procedure for evaluating policy against a set of criteria. Evaluation, even of efficiency criteria, is a normative process which requires explicit discussion of underlying value judgements, to derive specific answers to policy problems.

REFERENCES

BMJ editorial (1986) 'Government hypocrisy on drugs', *British Medical Journal* 292:712-13.

Central Statistical Office (1987) *United Kingdom National Accounts* (CSO Blue Book) London: HMSO.

Crain, M., Deaton, T., Holcombe, R., and Tollinson, R. (1977) 'Rational choice and the taxation of sin', *Journal of Public Economics* 8:239-45.

Department of Health and Social Security (1985) *Cooperation at the Community Level on Health Related Problems*, Memorandum to the House of Lords Select Committee on the European Community, London: HMSO.

Dunbar, G. C. and Morgan, D. D. V. (1987) 'The changing pattern of alcohol consumption in England and Wales 1978-85', *British Medical Journal* 295:807-10.

General Household Survey (1986) *The General Household Survey 1984*, London: HMSO.

Godfrey, C. and Powell, M. (1987) 'Making economic sense of social cost studies of alcohol and tobacco', in *The Cost of Alcohol, Drugs and Tobacco to Society, Papers and Abstracts*, Institute for Preventive and Social Psychiatry, Erasmus University Rotterdam.

Green College Consensus (1987) 'Passive smoking in the workplace – nuisance or risk?', *Community Medicine* 9(3):209-15.

Health and Lifestyle Survey (1987) London: Health Promotion Research Trust.

International Classification of Diseases (1979) 9th edn, Geneva: WHO Offset Publications.

Ledermann, S. (1956) 'Alcool, Alcoolisme, Alcoolisation', Institut Nationale d'Etudes Demographiques, Cahier no. 29, Paris: Presses Universitaires de France.

Leedham, W. (1987) 'Data note 10. Alcohol, tobacco and public opinion', *British Journal of Addiction* 82:935-40.

Littlechild, S. C. and Wiseman, J. (1986) 'The political economy of restriction of choice', *Public Choice* 51:161-72.

McDonnell, R. and Maynard, A. (1985a) 'Counting the cost of alcohol: gaps in epidemiological knowledge', *Community Medicine* 7:4-17.

McDonnell, R. and Maynard, A. (1985b) 'Estimation of life years lost from alcohol related preventive death', *Alcohol and Addiction* 20:435-43.

Maynard, A., Hardman, G., and Whelan, A. (1987) 'Data note 9. Measuring the social costs of addictive substances', *British Journal of Addiction* 82:701-6.

Royal College of General Practitioners (1986) *Alcohol: A Balanced View*, Report from General Practice 24, London: RCGP.

Royal College of Physicians (1983) *Health or Smoking? A Follow-up Report*, London: Pitman.

Royal College of Physicians (1987) *A Great and Growing Evil: The Medical Consequences of Alcohol Abuse*, London: Tavistock.

Royal College of Psychiatrists (1979) *Alcohol and Alcoholism*, London: Tavistock.

Royal College of Psychiatrists (1986) *Alcohol Our Favourite Drug*, London: Tavistock.

Tether, P. and Harrison, L. (1986) 'Data note 3. Alcohol-related fires and drownings', *British Journal of Addiction* 81:425-31.

Thorley, A. (1982) 'The effects of alcohol', in M. Plant (ed.) *Drinking and Problem Drinking*, London: Junction Books.

Varian, H. R. (1978) *Microeconomic Analysis*, New York: Norton.

Waller, J. A. (1986) On smoking and drinking and crashing', *New York State Journal of Medicine* 86(9):459-60.

Wilson, P. (1980) *Drinking in England and Wales*, London: HMSO.

World Health Organization (1985) *Strategies for Health for All in Europe: Regional Evaluation*, 35th Session of the Regional Committee [EUR/RC35/6].

Wright, S. J. (1987) 'Self ratings of health: the influence of age and smoking status and the role of different explanatory models', *Psychology and Health* 1(4):379-97.

Chapter Fourteen

The QALY
How can it be used?

CLAIRE GUDEX

THE DEVELOPMENT OF COST-UTILITY AND QALY CONCEPTS

Interest in health outcome measurement has grown steadily over the last few years. Although health economists are considered to be the main protagonists of work in this field, the impetus behind the original development of such concepts as the QALY came more from two other groups – the members of the medical profession and of health service management. Possibly by virtue of being a third party, health economists have been able to identify common goals of these independent and often opposing groups, and present these in a framework combining social, medical, and economic concepts. Despite common aspirations however, the two groups have very different philosophies on the aims of medical practice, inevitable given their different professional backgrounds.

Doctors have always been concerned with the effect of their treatment on patients. This stems mainly from altruism, but in addition there has always been a healthy awareness of the penalties of a poor outcome. These range from answering charges of negligence in a modern law court, to, in the seventeenth century, the loss of a prestigious position in a royal court. It was also wise to ensure the approval of one's peers – in the early days of the College of Physicians it was remarked that 'unauthorized practitioners were deemed worthy of punishment or otherwise, not as they killed or cured his Majesty's subjects, but as they were insolent or humble to the College' (King 1958). In comparison to a group such as health service management however, the prime focus for most medical practitioners is the individual patient, despite the widening of responsibility of some of the profession through the development of public health measures in the nineteenth century followed by the speciality of Community Medicine. From the intimate nature of the relationship between patient and doctor grew the notion of the doctor's responsibility to the patient, requiring in particular the confidentiality of patient information. The basic premise of a doctor's actions was, and continues to be, to provide as much treatment as is necessary, or indeed possible, to cure each patient.

The desire to maximize the effects of treatment for patients has led some doctors to become involved in studies assessing outcomes from health care. There is now a wide range of scales on which to measure this outcome, although most are clinically orientated and disease-specified, e.g. Hip Function Index, NIH Clinical Score for Cystic Fibrosis, Glasgow Coma Scale.

The pressure to monitor outcome does not only arise from within the patient-doctor relationship. There are growing demands on the health service from an increasingly health-conscious but also ageing population, and rising costs of health care, which create external pressures affecting everyone involved in the health care system. These pressures have been present for several decades but have become acute in the last ten years as public expenditure policies create an environment of scarce resources and competition for funding. Many doctors, particularly those working in government-funded hospitals, find themselves having to measure their performance against others in the same field and to prove the worth of their own work. This in itself may not create difficulties as it can be seen to be in the patient's best interest and in many cases there is genuine doubt as to the best method of treatment. However it is more foreign to a medical practitioner to be forced to consider economic consequences of his or her actions, especially when these considerations appear to undermine or even oppose medical ethics. Failure to treat a patient because of staff shortages, or because treatment is simply too costly, goes very much against the grain of basic medical tenets. In recent years lectures on health economics have been included in the curricula for medical schools, but for most doctors concepts such as cost-effectiveness and opportunity costs have little meaning or relevance.

In parallel with the growing funding problems faced by the health service, management is also having to alter its approach to decision making and to incorporate new ideas. There is a move towards greater accountability and an emphasis on cost-minimizing as well as cost-saving procedures. It is now generally accepted that the resources available to meet the demands of health care are limited. This forces difficult allocation decisions where resources must be split among competing uses. In contrast to clinical medicine, management is concerned with groups of patients, often numbered in thousands. It has to form priorities for allocating resources between different medical specialities, patients with different conditions and illnesses, population groups such as the elderly, neonates, and mentally handicapped, and even between primary and secondary health care. Traditional criteria have included mortality data, numbers of patients, costs, availability of staff and facilities, and also political importance. Decisions are often inconsistent however, and as yet, there is no systematic analysis of a set of standard criteria to allow decision makers to draw valid comparisons between alternative uses of resources. There is also a need for the inclusion of more relevant measures of patient outcome, in particular quality of survival.

From this discussion it is apparent that the organizations and individuals who actually make resource allocation decisions usually have varying objectives that need to be recognized and included in a more systematic framework. In an attempt to do this, an increasing number of researchers are using approaches such as cost-effectiveness and cost-benefit analyses to suggest guides for present and future decisions.

Any such analysis has two components. First the financial costs of developing or expanding a programme, second the benefits for the patient at whom it is aimed, measured in life years or QALYs.

The advantage of the QALY is that it combines effects on survival and morbidity in a single measure that reflects trade-offs between these two factors. It represents information that doctors and patients rely on, however implicitly, when a choice between alternative treatments is possible. Cost/QALY information is not being advocated as the only criterion upon which decisions should be made, but as an extra source of data to add to the information already used. It is a mechanism whereby the health aspirations of society can be incorporated into the decision processes of the health care system.

In the next section, some of the QALY research that has been carried out at the Centre for Health Economics is described, after a brief history of the QALY concept. The third section deals with the

220

main implications of the use of cost per QALY information in policy decisions, including both ethical and practical considerations.

HOW QALYS CAN BE USED: SOME EXAMPLES

The NHS provides a natural framework for the application of health economic analysis. Even so, although health authorities in the United Kingdom have been the first to assess the actual feasibility of incorporating QALYs into resource allocation decisions, the initial studies involving QALYs and their applications came from the United States.

Nearly twenty years ago, Herbert Klarman, Professor of Public Health Administration and of Political Economy at Johns Hopkins University, published with his colleagues results of a cost-effectiveness analysis applied to the treatment of Chronic Renal Disease (Klarman, O'Francis, and Rosenthal 1968). Since then, further research has been carried out on both conceptual and method-ological issues of QALYs, by several multidisciplinary groups in the United States and in Canada.

Torrance (1986) provides a useful review of much of this work, and it becomes apparent that the cost per QALY approach can be applied to a range of activities in the health care system. These include both primary and secondary health care, highly techno-logical procedures as well as community screening and preventive measures. There is considerable interest in the field, and with on-going research, more information is being generated on the methodology allowing refinement of techniques and more effective application.

The involvement in the field of QALY application of the Centre for Health Economics at York is therefore rather a recent one. As already indicated, however, it is the first group to test the practical feasibility of using QALYs to aid real-life resource allocation decisions. Only in this way can the advantages and implications of using QALYs be assessed and discussed by the different parties involved.

The North Western Regional Health Authority has been particu-larly interested in using QALYs in their decisions for resource allo-cation. In 1985-6 the Centre for Health Economics took part in a joint project with the primary aim of testing the feasibility of QALY data as one of the criteria in assessing bids for health care. If the data

were found to be useful, a system could then be devised for calculating and incorporating QALYs routinely into future bids.

Many of the major medical specialties are represented in the top
10 spenders of the Regional Speciality Development Fund (RSDF),
and the services tend to be of high priority regionally and nationally,
and are often dramatically life-enhancing or life-saving. However,
they are also expensive and in the year 1986–7, the total bids against
the RSDF totalled £8.9m in the face of £1.7m available.

With such a range of medical procedures which affect people's
lives in very different ways, it is extremely difficult to compare the
merits of each bid in a systematic way. To allow such a comparison
cost/QALY data were calculated for several of these procedures.
The areas chosen came from regional specialties, partly because of
their high priority and cost, but also because there was more likely
to be well-documented literature on clinical trials. The selected bids
were those that were directly patient-related, so that outcome data
would be more directly accessible. The chosen treatments were
those related to: (a) end-stage renal disease (b) upper limb joint
replacement (c) surgery for scoliosis and (d) the use of a new drug in
the treatment of cystic fibrosis. Data on quality of life and survival
were collated from published literature, while the Health Authority
provided costing information.

Some of the results are shown in Table 14.1, which indicates the
relative benefits from a variety of procedures; it is evident that
different health care activities show very different cost-effectiveness.
To provide a sense of perspective, it should be noted that the average
level of GNP per head in Britain is about £5,000 per annum.

Continuous ambulatory peritoneal dialysis (CAPD) appears to be
the least cost-effective procedure. The QALY gain used here is that
expected for marginal patients who would be accepted into the
CAPD programme in the event of increased funding. These may be
elderly patients or those with medical complications. Their poorer
expectations of survival, combined with the high cost of CAPD,
make the cost/QALY very high. Hospital haemodialysis, and ceftaz-
idime treatment in cystic fibrosis are more cost-effective, but are still
expensive in terms of inputs required. At a much reduced cost are
kidney transplantation and shoulder joint replacement. These
would seem well worthwhile procedures in view of the benefits that
patients perceive themselves as receiving, and the lower costs
involved. It should be noted here, however, that the cost cited for

Table 14.1   Examples of cost per QALY for selected bids for funds in a
particular regional health authority

	QALYs gained per patient (discounted at 5%)	Annual cost per patient (£)	Total cost (discounted at 5%) (£)	Cost/ QALY (£)
CAPD (4 year survival)	3.4	12,866	45,676	13,434**
Hospital haemodialysis (8 year survival)	6.1	8,569	55,354	9,075**
Treatment of cystic fibrosis with cetfazidime (over 22 years)	0.4	250	3,290	8,255**
Kidney transplant (lasting 10 years)	7.4	10,452	10,452	1,413*
Shoulder joint replacement (lasting 10 years)	0.9	533	533	592*
Scoliosis surgery – idiopathic adolescent	1.2	3,143	3,143	2,619*
– neuromuscular illness	16.2	3,143	3,143	194*

*Represents one-off costs per case, and benefits discounted over life of case.
**Represents recurring annual costs and annual QALYs per case.
Source: Gudex (1986)

kidney transplantation does not include the cost of immuno-suppressant drug treatment which patients continue to receive for some time after the operation. At the bottom of the list, being the most cost-effective procedure, is scoliosis surgery for neuromuscular illness. This type of surgery confers a substantial improvement in quality of life for the patients involved and is also cheap. Surgery for idiopathic adolescent scoliosis does not do so well because of the less dramatic effects on quality of life and on survival.

The variation in results for scoliosis surgery, for example, emphasizes the importance of determining *precisely* what are the activities being compared and the characteristics of patients involved. The QALY figures cited in the table have been calculated by comparing the benefits with no treatment in all cases except for the treatment of cystic fibrosis, which was derived from the benefits of a new anti-biotic above current established treatment. Clearly results could differ if, for example, benefits of the new drug were compared with no treatment at all.

Similarly it is important to know the characteristics of patients. For a 50-year-old patient with renal failure, treatment by hospital haemodialysis may confer an extra 6.1 QALYs with a survival of 8 years. But if this patient had complications such as heart failure, a blocked fistula, or recurrent infections, with a resulting survival of only 2 years, the QALYs gained may only be 1.8.

The application of QALYs is not limited to regional specialities. Some preliminary work has been done by Williams (1986) on strategies for the prevention of coronary heart disease. Costs per QALY for 3 such strategies are indicated in Table 14.2, which shows that the counselling of patients by GPs to give up smoking could be a very cost-effective measure.

This sort of information would undoubtedly be of benefit to health authorities and others participating in decisions for resource allocation. Assumptions and estimates are necessary at present to fill the gaps in knowledge of benefits and costs. However the final cost/QALY figures show such variations in magnitude that even a crude calculation could give an idea of cost-effectiveness.

ETHICAL AND PRACTICAL IMPLICATIONS OF USING QALYs IN POLICY DECISIONS

It is suggested that cost per QALY data should be added to information already considered in funding decisions within the health

Table 14.2 Cost per QALY for 3 strategies open to GPs for the prevention of coronary heart disease*

Strategy	Approximate cost per QALY
Advice to stop smoking	Less than £180
Action to control severe hypertension	£1,700 (or perhaps somewhat lower)
Action to control total serum cholesterol levels	£1,700 (or perhaps slightly higher)

*Based on screening 1000 male patients over 40 years of age consulting their GPs for any reason whatever.
For details see Williams (1986)

care sector, to form a more reliable and more explicit basis on which to make decisions. It is suggested that those procedures or activities which are most cost-effective, i.e. produce the most benefit for a given cost, should be developed or supplied first. Activities conferring less general benefit should be given a lower priority. This does not mean that such activities would never receive funding. In any new development of a service, and in many fields of research, initial costs can be very high, and health benefits are not always immediately obvious. These areas will continue to require funding, but it would be recommended that attention is first drawn to areas of more obvious need. Funding here would be of more immediate benefit to receivers, and also probably to the health service in the long term. Such activities, which often involve low technology and are community or primary care orientated, tend to be easily overlooked in the current preference for cure-orientated, high technology medicine.

A method such as this for assessing bids in a more systematic way, must help the Health Service to become more efficient. It will do this not only by placing an emphasis on activities which produce more benefit per cost, and also identifying areas of need, but also by encouraging participants to use and clarify outcome measurements. These are visibly lacking in the present system. Outcome data would provide feedback to assess the effectiveness of the health system, and would probably increase the participation of the general population in the health care field. This latter effect would certainly be desirable as it is this population for which the health system was established.

The use of cost per QALY information in policy decisions does however, raise some important ethical and practical issues which need to be recognised and discussed.

Ethical implications

When QALYs are used in resource allocation decisions, *choices between patient groups* competing for medical care are made explicit. There is an implication that some patients will be refused or not offered treatment in preference to others. These concerns have not been traditionally part of a doctor's way of thinking and therefore it may be difficult for some of the medical fraternity to accept the QALY concept. It is expected that a doctor does all that is possible for patients to maximize their health. However, it must be realized that such choices have always been made, although not formally identified. Doctors who treat private patients do so at the expense of public patients, those who work in cities do so at the expense of the rural community, those who do heart transplants do so at the expense of patients on a waiting list for pacemakers, and so on. Choices are being made all the time and priorities are being set, and decisions are now becoming more difficult with the increasing demands on limited resources within the health system.

The real question then, is not whether these decisions need to be made, but *on what basis* are they being made? And are the decisions equally fair to all patient groups? Are there any patient groups who consistently receive less or poorer health care, or who consistently suffer poorer health? It may be considered that as members of society, doctors have a responsibility to society as a whole and not only to individual patients, despite the fact that when faced with an ill patient it is painful to realize that treatment of this patient may be at the expense of another. There is a commitment to ensure that the choices made are the efficient and humane ones, and are not based merely on political pressure or the quest for technological advancement. With their expert knowledge of treatment and outcome, doctors have a significant role to play in this decision making. They are responsible for so much of the processes within the health care system, that they can make a valuable contribution to the decision making process.

Whose values should count when health states are being compared?

The question of who should be asked to do the valuations is open to debate. Responses from a large sample (500 or even 1,000 subjects) of the general population could be used, with the argument that the health care system is set up for the general population which therefore has a right to have its own value of life represented.

Health workers could be asked because they are the ones delivering health care, and have the closest and widest contact with patients, and hence may claim to be the people best able to reflect patients' views (other than patients themselves). Or perhaps politicians and health authority officers should be asked as they are the ones charged with priority setting, resource allocation, and the planning and administration of health care. Then of course, perhaps only people already suffering from particular disabilities should be the evaluators because only they know how their Quality of Life (QoL) has been changed and to what degree. Sackett and Torrance (1978) presented results indicating differences between valuations given by healthy volunteers and by patients. The valuations of the latter were themselves dependent on the length of illness.

Despite the small number of respondents, an analysis by Rosser and Kind (1978) of valuations given by various subjects, shows a surprising and encouraging consistency among respondents. It was noted however, that doctors placed more emphasis on distress, while patients felt disability to be more important.

Clearly, further study is required to determine how different subject groups value QoL. If the resulting valuation sets are significantly different, the question of whose values to use becomes crucial, as do sensitivity analyses of cost per QALY data. Then the discussion as to whose values count (if it is not to be an aggregated valuation set) should not be confined to the realm of health economics, but should be much wider as it brings into question some quite basic beliefs about the philosophy of the health care system.

Are people 'equal'?

One of the premises upon which the current calculation of QALYs is based, is that one year of healthy life expectancy is of equal value no matter who gets it, and other health states are valued relatively to this 'standard' unit of value by each individual whose valuations have equal weight. It is therefore assumed that the value of an individual remains the same throughout his or her life. The NHS has the basic tenet of equity, with equal distribution of and access to health for every member of the population. So it could be assumed that every individual has an equal value to society. However some people contest this assumption and suggest that perhaps an individual's value to society changes throughout his or her life.

The general population is often seen as a source of human capital. Patients are then assessed in terms of their actual or potential value to society with respect to income. It is thought that those patients who are likely to be useful economically to society should receive a greater input of health benefits with a view to maximizing their contribution to society. This view discriminates against several groups, in particular housewives, the elderly, and the mentally or physically handicapped. It tends not to take into account a person's past contribution to society.

On the basis of results from a recent survey (Wright 1986) perhaps the quality of life for certain age groups should be weighted higher relative to the quality of life for some other age groups. It appears that both males and females feel that the most important times to be in good health during their lives include early parenthood, infancy, when setting up a first home (males), at the peak of earning capacity (males), and when caring for elderly relatives (females). From these results it could be suggested that quality of life ratings should be weighted in favour of infants and adults up to about 50 years old. This scale however would also discriminate against the elderly.

If society does hold a view of differential value of individuals, it would be quite feasible to include such a weighting system into the calculation of QALYs, rather than the current judgement that 1 QALY is of equal value to everybody.

Practical implications

Since they are calculated from survival and quality of life data that clinicians and patients consider, QALYs represent information that is already included at one level in health care decisions. However during most QALY application exercises, it rapidly becomes apparent that little of the outcome data available is in a form that allows inclusion in the calculations.

In addition to detailed data on costs, and number and characteristics of patients, one also needs to know the implications of treatment for the patient, in terms of both life expectancy and quality of survival (currently represented by disability and distress). Most cost per QALY applications require the comparison of health benefits of a proposed new treatment against those of the traditional or established treatment, or against no treatment at all. As it stands at present, the onus would be on management to ensure that this data is gathered from various sources, in particular from the clinicians involved. This in turn would require more extensive communication and cooperation between management and hospital staff, which may slow down the process of resource allocation decisions until participants became more accustomed to the approach.

Further practical implications of using QALYs concern the methodology itself, in particular the measurement of health-related quality of life. These issues are clearly important and relevant to the concept of QALYs and are discussed elsewhere (see Kind and Loomes and MacKenzie in this volume).

There is debate over the rate of discounting which should be used in QALY calculation, and indeed, some researchers are of the opinion that QALYs should not be discounted at all. In most cost-utility studies, QALYs are discounted at the same rate as the costs, and the rate chosen is usually the Treasury public discount rate. It is thus assumed that, as with future costs, future benefits are worth less than immediate ones.

To date however, there has been little investigation into the way future benefits are perceived, and whether benefits in terms of QoL and years of survival can be treated in a similar way to costs. Until more is known about these issues, details of the discounting rates should be made explicit in any cost per QALY calculations, allowing different rates to be used if required.

SUMMARY

The development of the QALY concept is an attempt to provide a fairer and more systematic way of setting priorities in the health care system. The additional information it represents widens the criteria on which decisions are made, and it brings this information out into the open for public debate.

There is no doubt that the further research being carried out into the methodology and application of QALYs will broaden the base of experience in the field, which will in turn lead to more effective application of QALYs and to better health care management.

REFERENCES

Gudex, C. (1986) 'QALYs and their use by the health service', Discussion Paper no. 20, Centre for Health Economics, University of York.

King, L. S. (1958) *Medical World of the Eighteenth Century*, Chicago: University of Chicago Press.

Klarman, H. .E., O'Francis, J., and Rosenthal, G. D. (1968) 'Cost-effectiveness analysis applied to the treatment of chronic renal disease', *Medical Care* 6(1):48-54.

Rosser, R. M. and Kind, P. (1978) 'A scale of valuations of states of illness: is there a social consensus?' *International Journal of Epidemiology* 7(4): 347-58

Sackett, D. L. and Torrance, G. W. (1978) 'The utility of different health states', *Journal of Chronic Diseases* 31:697-704.

Torrance, G. W. (1986) 'Measurement of health state utilities for economic appraisal', *Journal of Health Economics* 5(1):1-30.

Williams, A. (1986) 'Screening for risk of CHD: is it a wise use of resources?', in M. Oliver, M. Ashley-Miller, and D. Wood (eds) *Strategy for Screening for Risk of Coronary Heart Disease*, Wiley.

Wright, S. (1986) 'Age, sex and health: a summary of findings from the York Health Evaluation Survey', Discussion Paper no. 15, Centre for Health Economics, University of York.

Chapter Fifteen

TREATING AIDS
Is it ethical to be efficient?

ALISON EASTWOOD and ALAN MAYNARD

INTRODUCTION

The National Health Service (NHS) in the UK is faced with virtual unlimited demand for its services, but is resources are limited. As a consequence, choices have to be made and priorities determined. Resource allocation in the NHS is ideally determined by the benefit principle, that is, resources are allocated, regardless of the individuals' willingness and ability to pay, to those patients who will benefit most from treatment. The benefit of health care expenditure is its effect on the subsequent length and quality of life. One measure of this outcome is the quality adjusted life year (or QALY). In this paper we have assumed that the objective of the NHS is to maximize the production of QALYs or some other outcome (or benefit) measure, because by so doing total benefits derived from the Service's finite budget are maximized. Therefore the principle for allocating scarce resources is the patient's capacity to benefit and treatment should go to those patients whose care produces most QALYs (or some other outcome measure). This approach is utilitarian, in that it creates the greatest benefit for the greatest number.

The acquired immune deficiency syndrome (AIDS) is a virulent disease of pandemic proportions. The implications of its spread are far-reaching in terms of mortality, morbidity, and the opportunity costs of treatment. In this paper, the implications of the treatment of people with AIDS in the UK are examined. In the first section various aspects of the etiology of AIDS and data collection in the UK are examined. A number of forecasts have been made for future levels of the disease and these are described in the second section together with the current estimates of survival time of people with AIDS and the estimated costs of treatment. In the third section the

231

efficiency and cost implications of the treatment of people with AIDS examined and the difficult trade-offs between efficiency and treatment are indicated.

HISTORY AND ETIOLOGY OF AIDS AND UK DATA ON AIDS

Etiology of AIDS

The acquired immune deficiency syndrome came to public attention in the UK in the early 1980s. It is difficult to pinpoint the first diagnosed cases because of lack of knowledge at the time, but it is possible that retrospective diagnoses could go back into the 1970s. AIDS is the most severe consequence of infection with human immunodeficiency virus (HIV) and to date there is no cure for the disease. The presence of HIV antibodies in blood can be tested for, but is no guide to the severity of exposure or likely prognosis.

Wells (1986) describes two stages of infection; the acute stage in which antibody development occurs, in which the patient may have a feeling of general malaise, and the chronic stage which can lead to Persistent Generalized Lymphadenopathy (PGL) or AIDS-related complex (ARC), although the individual may remain asymptomatic. It is estimated that 35-45 per cent of all HIV patients (that is, patients infected with HIV) develop PGL or ARC. Prognosis for individuals with PGL can be quite good, but for ARC patients there is a high risk that they will contract the full AIDS symptoms. Figure 15.1 shows the possible routes which HIV infection can take.

At present, about half of the total number of reported AIDS cases are still alive. This implies a case fatality rate of approximately 50 per cent. However, to date, nobody has recovered from AIDS and so the overall long term mortality rate is 100 per cent.

Different groups of society have been highlighted as 'high risk' groups in which HIV infection is more prevalent. The figures in Table 15.1 show the prevalence of HIV-positive people among different 'risk' groups. It is generally assumed that homosexual men are most 'at risk' from HIV infection mainly through sexual transmission. Haemophiliacs have also been open to HIV infection through use of contaminated blood products, although this method of transmission is now very unlikely due to the heat treat-

232

Figure 15.1 Possible routes of HIV infection

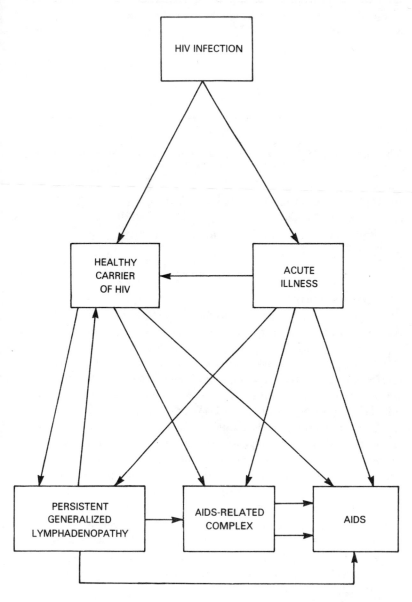

Source: Wells (1986).

Table 15.1   Prevalence of anti-HTLV-III in UK risk groups
1984–5

Risk group	Number tested	Number anti-HTLV-III positive[2] (%)
Homosexual men	4,035	860 (21)
Haemophiliacs	1,847	577 (31)
Drug abusers	239	24 (10)
Unspecified[1]	6,605	722 (11)
Total	12,726	2,183 (17)

Source: Jesson et al. 1986
1. This group consists mainly of homosexual men.
2. The terminology 'HTLV-III' has been replaced by 'HIV' and so 'anti-HTLV-III' corresponds to HIV antibody positive or simply 'HIV positive' in the main text.

ment of blood products such as factor VIII and IX. The other main 'high risk' group is intravenous drug abusers (IVDAs) where transmission can occur through contaminated needles.

Data sources

The Department of Health and Social Security (DHSS) publish data, prepared by the Communicable Disease Surveillance Centre (CDSC) and Communicable Disease (Scotland) Unit (CD(Scotland)U). These data provide monthly figures of reported AIDS cases and deaths and quarterly figures of HIV infection (DHSS 1987a) by 'region' and by 'patient characteristic'. The figures must be viewed with caution as it is likely that both under reporting and late reporting occur. The HIV figures relate only to positive antibody test results and do not reflect the large number of people unaware of their seropositivity, or infected people who have not as yet developed antibodies. The reported AIDS figures may be underestimates for reasons such as the failure to diagnose AIDS and unwillingness by GPs to report cases or deaths to avoid causing distress to their patients. However, to date there are no alternative data and this situation is unlikely to change in the near future. The CDSC and CD(Scotland)U request that relevant cases are reported to them in confidence, but AIDS has not been classified as a communicable disease and so reporting is not compulsory. The Health Education Authority is setting up a dedicated unit on AIDS and intends to introduce a national database, but this is still in its infancy.

Up to the end of September 1987 there had been 1,067 diagnoses of AIDS cases reported in the UK and 605 deaths, with a reported 7,557 HIV antibody positive persons (see Figure 15.2). The level of HIV infection is measured by the number of positive results to HIV antibody tests, the true level in the population will be much greater – current estimates put the figure around 40,000 people infected with HIV in the UK (DHSS 1987a:87/346), although estimates range from 30,000 to 100,000 (Wilkie 1987).

FORECASTS OF FUTURE RATES OF HIV INFECTION AND AIDS AND LENGTH OF SURVIVAL

Actual and predicted cases

It is difficult to make accurate predictions of future numbers of AIDS cases and HIV infection because of the limitations of the data. In the UK, AIDS surveillance was introduced at the beginning of 1982, and HIV reporting began in 1984. Thus there are about five years of incomplete figures on AIDS and approximately three on HIV infection. However there have been attempts at predicting future numbers of AIDS cases and at modelling the prevalence of both HIV and AIDS. Tables 15.2a and 15.2b provide a summary of the various predictions and the 'actual' numbers published by the DHSS.

Rees (1987a) uses data reported by Peterman *et al.* (1985), a sample of 144 cases of transfusion-related HIV infection where the individuals have gone on to develop AIDS and an exact time of infection can be determined. He assumes that the development of AIDS is described by a normal distribution with mean incubation of 15 years (i.e. the average time from infection to development of AIDS is 15 years) and that all HIV infections will eventually lead to AIDS. He estimates 23,646 new infections in 1985 with a total number of 109,288 infections up to the end of 1985. Rees also notes that if the log-normal distribution fits the data better than the normal distribution, then the number of AIDS cases would rise more sharply in the early years and peak sooner. However, there have been a number of responses to Rees and these assert that the mean incubation period is closer to 5 years than 15 years (Lui *et al.*

Figure 15.2   Cumulative AIDS cases in the UK

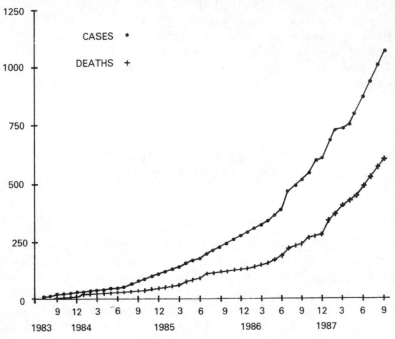

Source: personal communication DHSS.

1986; Iversen and Engen 1986; Barton 1987; Beal 1987; Costagliola and Downs 1987).

May and Anderson (1987) analyse the transmission dynamics of HIV infection using mathematical models. They believe the key parameter to be the reproductive rate of infection, which they define as the average number of secondary infections produced by one infected individual in the early stages of the epidemic. To maintain the epidemic, this reproduction rate must be greater than unity. The reproduction rate is dependent on the rate of acquiring new part-ners, the probability of transmitting the infection and the average length of infectiousness. In the early stages of the epidemic the frac-tion of the population who are infected will rise exponentially. In later stages the increase should become linear rather than expo-nential. May and Anderson assume that the incubation period follows a Weibull distribution, with mean 4-5 years. Since the

236

Table 15.2a   Predicted and actual numbers of new AIDS cases

	1984	1985	1986	1987	1988
McEvoy and Tillett (1985 estimate)		144	336	785	837
McEvoy and Tillett (1986 estimate)		240	550	1,300	3,000
Mortimer (estimate)	59	187	620	1,095	1,847
DHSS (reported actuals)	77	167	335	457[1]	

Table 15.2b   Predicted and actual numbers of AIDS deaths (in each year)

	1983	1984	1985	1986	1987	1988
Wilkie (estimate)[2] (i)	0	23	77	167	334	652
(ii)	0	11	39	86	173	337
(iii)	0	38	117	235	458	892
DHSS (reported actuals)	11	35	81	153	325[1]	

1. Up to 30 September 1987.
2. Wilkie obtained seven different projections by varying the parameters of his standard Basis model. The three projections given in the table are:
    (i)   the standard Basis;
    (ii) the minimum projection of deaths for the period 1983–8;
    (iii) the maximum projection of deaths for the period 1983–8.
    Sources: DHSS 1987a; Wilkie 1987; McEvoy and Tillett 1985, 1986; Mortimer 1985; DHSS, personal communication

fraction of HIV infected people who develop AIDS is unknown, it is difficult to obtain a prediction of the incidence of AIDS. It is difficult to judge whether the epidemic will increase or decrease if the fraction of HIV carriers who go on to develop AIDS increases. It is possible that the epidemic will decrease if the major cause of transmission is by unknowing asymptomatic HIV carriers. Also, nothing is known about the infectiousness of those who are HIV carriers but do not develop AIDS. They may stay infectious for a long time and therefore have the potential to transmit the disease to a large number of people.

Anderson *et al.* (1987) attempt to predict the minimum size of the AIDS epidemic in the UK (by assuming all transmission ceases at the end of 1986), and obtain predictions ranging from 5,822 to 24,985 AIDS deaths by 1994 depending on the values of the parameters used (incubation periods of 4.3 and 8 years and probabilities that HIV infection will lead to AIDS ranging from 0.3 to 1.0). Their results show that even the minimum size of the epidemic is difficult to predict. The predictions are very sensitive to changes in the parameters (dropping the assumption that transmission ends in 1986 leads to a prediction of 63,035 deaths by 1994).

Medley *et al.* (1987) utilize a sample of 297 people with AIDS infected via blood transfusions in the US, and find age-related differences in mean (and median) incubation periods. This shows that the incubation period is shortest for children and longest for adults under the age of 60. However the shorter incubation period in elderly individuals could be related to a higher mortality rate following transfusion (unrelated to HIV infection). Thus more elderly people could die before AIDS develops. The authors voice the usual caveats about the data and analyse the fit of various simple mathematical forms to explain the growth in the number of infected individuals who will go on to develop AIDS. They conclude that exponential growth fits better than linear growth for infections via blood transfusions. The doubling time of the exponential model is approximately one year although the doubling time in children seems to be somewhat higher (1.3 years compared with 1.08 years for adults). There is a difference between male and female incubation periods, the former being shorter on average (mean 5.62, median 5.50 years) than the latter (mean 8.77, median 8.36 years).

Wilkie (1987) takes an actuarial approach to the future incidence of AIDS cases in the UK and examines the implications of the disease for actuarial work for pension funds and insurance companies. He assumes that all infected individuals will eventually die of AIDS if they do not die of something else first. The population is split into two groups 'clear' and 'at risk' where movement can occur as people adjust their behaviour from 'at risk,' to 'clear'. The model used by Wilkie is elaborate and dependent on a number of parameters and simplifying assumptions to arrive at varying projections of future deaths from AIDS. In each of the various projections the number of deaths reaches a peak and then declines to an approximately level number. The results range from a peak of 18,390 deaths from AIDS in the year 2000 up to a peak of 89,570 in 1999. Similarly the predicted number at which deaths 'level' out ranges from 3,800 to 15,200.

The limitations of the available data must be borne in mind when assessing predictions about the future level of AIDS and HIV infection. One major problem is that it is not possible to test the validity of the predictions with such a small data set. In the UK data have only been available for about 5 years in total and those for the first few years are very limited. Even now reporting is incomplete and this problem is unlikely to change in the short run. Some of the variables which are useful in describing the disease are very difficult to measure or incorporate into a mathematical/statistical model. For example, it is difficult to obtain precise details of sexual behaviour or the extent to which attitudes and behaviour are changing as information about HIV infection and AIDS becomes more widespread. Another problem is that many of the predictions are based on data which refer to transfusion-related HIV infection and AIDS cases. However, it is quite possible that rate of infection, incubation period and other relevant variables will depend upon the method of transmission, sex, age, and other such factors. In this situation the picture obtained from transfusion-related cases will not reflect the overall picture.

Length of survival

The most comprehensive study to date of the length of survival of people with AIDS in the UK is that of Marasca and McEvoy (1986). They carried out survival analysis on 168 AIDS cases reported to the CDSC and CD(Scotland)U up to 1 June 1985 (96 per cent of the total reported cases). The cases were categorized into four groups according to the mode of presentation, and the results obtained are given in Table 15.3.

The conclusions from this analysis provide a crude fatality rate for AIDS cases of 55 per cent and an average (median) survival time of 13.5 months. The most common mode of presentation was Pneumocystis carinii pneumonia (PCP) and the least common was Kaposis' sarcoma. People presenting with Kaposis' sarcoma had the longest median survival time whilst those with both Kaposis' sarcoma and PCP had the worst prognosis. The authors found no clear reasons for the differences in survival time.

McEvoy and Tillett (1985) in their analysis of 108 AIDS cases reported up to the end of 1984, estimated the death rate in the calendar year of presentation at 28 per cent. The estimated death rate in the calendar year after the year of presentation is 55 per cent. However, estimated rates for subsequent years are not calculable

Table 15.3   Length of survival of people with AIDS classified by presenting disease

Disease category		Median survival time (months)	Number of patients	Number dead (%)	Mean age (years)	75% patients dead (months)
(i)	Kaposis' sarcoma	21.2	44	21 (48)	38.5	44
(ii)	PCP	12.5	69	39 (57)	40.1	22
(iii)	Other opportunistic infection	13.3	43	24 (56)	35.7	NA
(iv)	Kaposis' sarcoma and PCP	6.6	12	9 (75)	36.0	10
	Total	13.5	168	93 (55)	38.0	28

Source: Marasca and McEvoy (1986)

since the number of survivors is too small.

Rees (1987b) took a sample of 63 people with AIDS at four London hospitals diagnosed as having AIDS between 1 January 1984 and 30 June 1985, 11 of whom were still alive in February 1987. From this analysis Rees found a mean survival time of over 400 days (13.2 months) and a mean length of inpatient stay of 90-100 days. The mean case has perhaps 4 spells in hospital with the length of time between spells declining significantly as death approaches. These figures assume a mean survival time from AIDS diagnosis of 265 days for the 52 people who had died and 771 days for the 11 people who were still alive. From his results, Rees suggests that it may be the case that mean survival time is increasing through time, although there is not enough information to determine whether this is true or not.

Since these articles were published the drug zidovudine (Retrovir)[1] has been licensed and is now used in the treatment of AIDS patients. Patients receiving the drug experience improved length of survival. In a double-blind, placebo-controlled trial in the USA (Fischl *et al.* 1987), it was found that the projected probability of 24-week survival was significantly greater for patients receiving Retrovir than for patients receiving the placebo (0.98 and 0.78 respectively). Conversely, the projected probability of opportunistic infection in the 24-week study period was significantly smaller for patients receiving Retrovir than for patients receiving the placebo (0.28 and 0.43 respectively).

To date, therefore, a 'guestimate' for the average length of survival is approximately 13 months, with a range of 6.6 months to 21.2 months (Marasca and McEvoy, 1987) depending on the mode of presentation.

Costs estimates per person

There have been few published attempts to cost AIDS (or HIV infection) in the UK. As for the epidemiological estimates there is very little information and care regimes are continually changing as different methods of treatment are developed. The introduction of Retrovir has significantly increased the cost of care. Adler (1987) has estimated a cost per annum of £6,600 to maintain one patient on Retrovir (depending on dosage and tolerance levels).

Johnson et al. (1986) examined 33 AIDS cases treated in Bloomsbury district hospital up to the end of June 1985, and estimated the total cost of lifetime care at £6,838 for each of the 16 patients who died during the period of analysis. They estimate a comprehensive service in the Bloomsbury district at £287,000 capital costs and £338,000 revenue costs for 1986–7. These costs relate to current hospital costs and ignore any increase in marginal costs that might result if more intensive nursing or new inpatient facilities were required. They also ignore all costs of community health, voluntary, and social services.

The one attempt that has been made to estimate the cost of comprehensive lifetime treatment of people with AIDS when care is community based was made by Cunningham and Griffiths (1987). They used data on patients presenting at St Marys Hospital, London with AIDS to December 1986 and estimate an average survival time of one year. They found a total lifetime cost of £20,805 for people not receiving Retrovir and £27,055 for people receiving Retrovir. The resource implications both directly (in terms of the drug costs) and indirectly (in terms of care during enhanced survival) are severe.

Costs to the NHS

Assuming Cunningham and Griffiths' (1987) estimate of lifetime costs of people with AIDS, the financial burden on the NHS can be estimated. Using McEvoy and Tillett's (1986) forecast of 1,300 new

AIDS cases in 1987 and 3,000 in 1988, and adjusting to account for late reporting (58 per cent of cases in 1985 were reported after November 1986), we might expect first reported figures of approximately 800 in 1987 and 2,000 in 1988 (assuming that retrospective reporting will diminish somewhat). Table 15.4 shows the possible total costs of treating these people. The figures are very rough and should be treated with caution (all cases are assumed to occur at the beginning of each year), but give some idea of the possible magnitude. If people with AIDS receiving Retrovir are included in the calculations the costs would be higher.

These calculations can be compared with those of Stuttaford (1987) who estimated that 'the virus' will cost the state more than £63m in 1988, although this may well be an underestimate as it assumes that only 10–20 per cent of infected people will go on to develop AIDS. Current estimates are that this proportion is higher (30–75 per cent). Our cost estimates are very sensitive to the assumptions used, but provide some guide to the magnitude of the problem.

One major problem is that the geographical incidence of HIV infection and AIDS amongst the population is uneven. Figure 15.3 shows the regional distribution of AIDS cases in England at the end of September 1987. From these figures it is apparent that 79 per cent of all AIDS cases were reported in London, 47 per cent in North West Thames and 20 per cent in North East Thames Regional Health Authorities. As reported in *New Scientist* (1987) the Government has allocated £1.6m this year to pay for Retrovir, £1m of these funds went to North West Thames Region, which also received an

Table 15.4 Estimated costs of people with AIDS to the NHS in 1988

| | Percentage receiving Retrovir | | | |
	100%	75%	50%	0%
People not receiving Retrovir (20,805 per person, per annum)	—	£13m	£26m	£52m
People receiving Retrovir (27,055 per person, per annum)	£68m	£51m	£34m	—
Total cost of all people	£68m	£64m	£60m	£52m

Assumes 2,500 people requiring treatment in 1988; approximately 2,000 new people in 1988 and 500 survivors from 1987.
Source: Authors' calculations using data from McEvoy and Tillett 1986 and Cunningham and Griffiths 1987

extra £2.5m towards the care of people with AIDS. In fact the region is spending about £6m, £2.5m more than the budget allows for and clearly this money must be raised from somewhere. It is also unknown whether these additional government monies will continue to be forthcoming or whether authorities will be expected to make provisions for Retrovir from their drug allocations.

If we take the cost-benefit approach to the problem, total benefit maximization requires that we examine not just cost but both the benefit (prolonged life, but to an unknown extent and possibly deteriorating quality) and the cost for each person with AIDS. More information is needed on the effects of the drug Retrovir in terms of quality of life, as there seems to be some division between doctors on the importance of the possible, very unpleasant, side effects. We estimate the cost to be up to £27,055 per annum for people treated with Retrovir.

EFFICIENCY AND COST IMPLICATIONS OF AIDS TREATMENT

Resource consequences

The resource consequences of HIV infection and subsequent AIDS are clearly very significant. It is unknown, as yet, exactly how large a problem it will become in future years, but current estimates imply the situation will worsen before it improves. It will prove a significant burden on NHS resources and to the extent that the government does not provide extra funds the burden will result in 'routine' NHS patients being deprived of care. The problem is how should such services be prioritized? Who should live and who should die in what degree of pain and discomfort?

Opportunity cost

The opportunity cost of treatment of AIDS patients is considerable (especially when treatment includes prescribing Retrovir) and the treatment is palliative not curative. Wells (1986) compares the cost of treatment of people with AIDS with: £4,732 for cardiac valve replacement, £5,915 for coronary artery graft, and £7,098 for first-year costs of renal transplant.

Figure 15.3   Cumulative AIDS cases in England by region of report

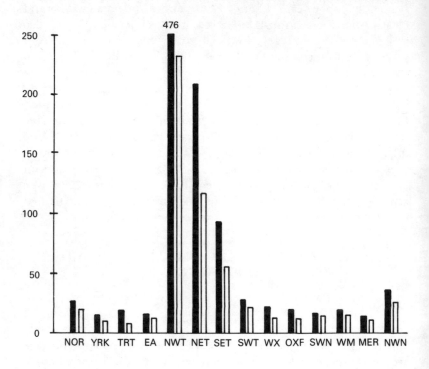

NOR – Northern
YKR – Yorkshire
TRT – Trent
EA – East Anglian
NWT – North West Thames
NET – North East Thames
SET – South East Thames
SWT – South West Thames
WX – Wessex
OXF – Oxford
SWN – South Western
WM – West Midlands
MER – Mersey
NWN – North Western

CASES

DEATHS

Source: DHSS (1987a).

Table 15.5   UK data on costs and QALYs

GP advice to stop smoking	167
Pacemaker implantation for atrioventricular heart block	700
Hip replacement	750
Valve replacement for aortic stenosis	900
CABG for severe angina with LMD	1,040
CABG for severe angina with 3VD	1,270
CABG for moderate angina with LMD	1,330
GP control of hypertension	1,700
GP control of total serum cholesterol	1,700
CABG for severe angina with 2VD	2,800
CABG for moderate angina with 3VD	2,400
CABG for mild angina with LMD	2,520
Kidney transplant	3,200
Breast cancer screening	3,309
Heart transplant	5,000
Hospital haemodialysis	14,000

Sources: Department of Health and Social Security (1987b) Williams (1985, 1986)

All of these treatments should significantly improve survival and quality of life. In comparison, £20,805 is the cost of providing palliative care for people with AIDS (without the drug Retrovir) with an estimated average survival time of approximately one year (_New Scientist_ 1987). In Table 15.5 we provide cost per QALY data for various treatments in the UK. These figures can be compared with the cost per QALY for people with AIDS. Clearly treating people with AIDS has a high cost per impaired QALY when compared to the crude cost per QALY estimate for treatment listed in Table 15.5.

Ethics and inefficiency

The treatment of people with AIDS, especially with Retrovir, is inefficient in terms of the 'guestimated' costs per QALY set out in Table 15.5 and this conclusion highlights the clash of medical and social imperatives.

The individual clinician is trained to treat his or her patients provided care provides some benefit. The physician is committed, according to Emanuel (1988), to 'the help and betterment of other people – selflessly caring for the sick' (p. 1686). However, such behaviour obviously has opportunity costs: resources allocated to the treatment of people with AIDS are not available to provide beneficial treatments such as hip replacements for the elderly. For Emanuel (1988) such considerations run counter to ethical medical practice and lie in the domain of political decision making.

However Emanuel's position is one which is questioned increasingly by medical practitioners. Roach *et al.* (1988) address the question of whether a patient with asymptomatic HIV infection should be treated if he presents with prostatic cancer. They conclude that the potential benefits of treating such a patient are substantially greater than the risks to the surgeon of giving treatment. However if the patient had symptomatic AIDS with its poor prognosis, the benefits from surgery would be small, and the surgeon's risks significant. This benefit-risk approach to treatment choices ignores opportunity cost but identifies circumstances in which treatment of patients would not be provided.

Grimes (1988) discusses other circumstances in which treatment might not be provided by physicians. He addresses the question of whether patients who smoke should be referred for coronary artery bypass grafting and argues that doctors should treat such patients whether or not they smoke. However he infers that political decision making might lead to national rules which deprived such smokers of treatments whose potential benefits might be reduced by the use of tobacco.

So the medical perspective, (Roach *et al.* 1988), appears to be that it is unacceptable to deprive patients of care which provides benefits, even though the cost of care might be very high. Their position appears to be that cost-benefit trade-offs and rationing decisions are in the political domain.

The rationing problem affects all patients, not just those with AIDS. If the objective of the NHS is to maximize improvements in health, then resources should be allocated on the basis of greatest benefit (QALY) and least cost. The consequence of this rule, in terms of the guestimates in Table 15.5, is that patients with illnesses such as end stage renal failure and AIDS might be left untreated.

This approach was set out clearly by Bishop Montefiore (1987):

> If an illness is always terminal and drugs exist which may delay
> death but with serious side effects, there is little point in
> spending vast sums on them to the detriment of many people
> waiting in pain for routine treatment of other kinds.
> When people have to wait three or four years for a hip joint
> operation and there is only so much money within the National
> Health Service, there is not a good moral case for spending vast

sums on drugs which are not a cure and which can have devastating side effects.

There is clearly a clash between the individual ethic of the doctor, to treat all patients who present to him or her, and the social ethic of the economist, to treat only those patients whose benefit is greatest relative to cost. The utilitarian approach to this clash would be to assert that the individual ethic will not lead to the greatest happiness of the greatest number, that is the maximization of health care benefits from a given NHS budget, and that it is unethical to be inefficient. An ethical response, to the scarcity of resources in utilitarian terms, is that only efficiency is ethical. Such a conclusion would not be accepted by clinicians and if adopted by society's representatives, the politicians, would oblige them to act ethically in utilitarian terms but unethically in terms of their professional codes. Such conflicts are inherent in all health care decision making and are likely to be made more explicit with the onset of the AIDS epidemic.

NOTE

1 Retrovir is the brand name for the drug zidovudine. However, it was first introduced as azidothymidine with the brand name AZT. It is still often referred to as AZT.

REFERENCES

Adler, M. W. (1987) 'Care for patients with HIV infection and AIDS', *British Medical Journal* 295:27–30.
Anderson, R. M., Medley, G. F., Blythe, S. P., and Johnson, A. M. (1987) 'Is it possible to predict the minimum size of the acquired immunodeficiency syndrome (AIDS) epidemic in the United Kingdom?' *Lancet* i:1073–5.
Barton, D. E. (1987) 'Striking the balance on AIDS', *Nature* 326:734.
Beal, S. (1987) 'On the sombre views of AIDS', *Nature* 328:673.
Costagliola, D. and Downs, A. M. (1987) 'Incubation time for AIDS', *Nature* 328:582.
Cunningham, D. and Griffiths, S. F. (1987) 'AIDS: counting the cost', *British Medical Journal* 295:921–2.
Department of Health and Social Security (1987a) Press Releases, HMSO.
    87/6, 8 Jan. 'Latest AIDS figures'.
    87/57, 9 Feb. 'Latest AIDS figures'.
    87/97, 9 Mar. 'Latest AIDS figures'.
    87/169, 10 Apr. 'New Quarterly figures on AIDS'.

87/193, 6 May 'Latest AIDS figures'.

87/222, 17 June 'Latest AIDS figures'.

87/245, 6 July 'Quarterly figures on AIDS'.

87/286, 10 Aug. 'Latest AIDS figures'.

87/311, 7 Sept. 'Latest AIDS figures'.

87/346, 5 Oct. 'Quarterly figures on AIDS'.

Department of Health and Social Security (1987b), *Breast Cancer Screening, Report to the Health Ministers of England, Wales, Scotland and Northern Ireland*, The Forrest Report, London: HMSO.

Emanuel, E. J. (1988) 'Do physicians have an obligation to treat patients with AIDS?', *New England Journal of Medicine* 318(25):1686–90.

Grimes, D. S. (1988) 'Should patients who smoke be referred for coronary artery by-pass grafting?', *Lancet* i:1157.

Fischl, M. A., Richman, D. D., Grieco, M. H., *et al.* (1987) 'The efficacy of Azidothymidine (AZT) in the treatment of patients with AIDS and AIDS-related complex', *New England Journal of Medicine* 317:185–91.

Iversen, O.-J. and Engen, S. (1986) 'Epidemiology of AIDS – statistical analysis' *Journal of Epidemiology and Community Health* 41:55–8.

Jesson, W. J., Thorp, R. W., Mortimer, P. P., and Oates, J. K., (1986) 'Prevalence of anti-HTLV-III in UK risk groups 1984/85', *Lancet* i:155.

Johnson, A. M., Adler, M. W., and Crown, J. M., (1986) 'The acquired immune deficiency syndrome and epidemic of infection with human immunodeficiency virus costs of care and prevention in an inner London district', *British Medical Journal* 293:489–92.

Lui, K.-J., Lawrence, D. N., Morgan, W. M., Peterman, T. A., Haverkos, H. W., and Bregman, D. J. (1986) 'A model-based approach for estimating the mean incubation period of transfusion-associated acquired immunodeficiency syndrome', *Proc. Natn. Acad. Sci. USA* 83:3051–5.

Marasca, G. and McEvoy, M. (1986) 'Length of survival of patients with acquired immune deficiency syndrome in the United Kingdom', *British Medical Journal* 292:1727–9.

May, R. M., and Anderson, R. M. (1987) 'Transmission dynamics of HIV infection', *Nature* 326:137–42.

McEvoy, M. and Tillett, H. (1985) 'Some problems in the prediction of future numbers of cases of the acquired immunodeficiency syndrome in the UK', *Lancet* ii:541–2.

McEvoy, M. and Tillett, H. (1986) 'Reassessment of predicted numbers of AIDS cases in the UK', *Lancet* ii:1104.

Medley, G. F., Anderson R. .M., Cox, D. R., and Billard, L. (1987) 'Incubation period of AIDS in patients infected via blood transfusion', *Nature* 328:719–21.

Montefiore, H. (1987) *The Times*, 27 August.

Mortimer, P. P. (1985) 'Estimating AIDS, UK', *Lancet* ii:1065.

New Scientist (1987) 1 October.

Peterman, T. A., Jaffe, H. W., Feorino, P. .M. *et al.* (1985) 'Transfusion-associated acquired immunodeficiency syndrome in the United States', *Journal of the American Medical Association* 254:2913–17.

Roach, P. J., Fleming, C., Hagen, M. D., and Parker, S. G. (1988) 'Prostatic cancer in a patient with asymptomatic HIV infection', *Medical Decision Making* 8(2):132–44.

Rees, M. (1987a) 'The sombre view of AIDS', *Nature* 326:343–5.

Rees, M. (1987b) 'Survival time, length of inpatient stay and hospital spells of UK AIDS patients', Unpublished.

Stuttaford, T. (1987) *The Times* (15 May).

Wells, N. (1986) *The AIDS virus: forecasting its impact*, London: Office of Health Economics.

Wilkie, D. (1987) *Preliminary Memorandum on AIDS*, Surrey: R. Watson & Sons.

Williams, A. (1985) 'Economics of coronary artery bypass grafting', *British Medical Journal* 291:326–9.

Williams, A. (1986) 'Screening for risk of coronary heart disease: is it a wise use of resources?' in M. Oliver, M. Ashley-Miller, and D. Wood, (eds) *Screening for Risk of Coronary Heart Disease*, Chichester: John Wiley & Sons.

AUTHOR INDEX

AUTHOR INDEX

251

SUBJECT INDEX